To Dr. Arlene,
A great friend
and a great woman!
Joan

TEXTBOOK ON

Chiropractic & Pregnancy

Joan Fallon, D.C.

INTERNATIONAL CHIROPRACTORS ASSOCIATION
Arlington, Virginia 22201

Project Editor: *Molly Rangnath*

Illustrator: *Joy Marlowe*

Designer: *Todd Dawson, Tripplaar & Associates*

Cover Design: *David Pfeiffer*

Library of Congress Catalog Card Number: 94-79060
ISBN 1-886190-00-3

FIRST EDITION

Printed in the United States.

Table of Contents

Introduction

This book was written with the intention of helping provide quality chiropractic care to the pregnant woman. It is not designed to be a substitute for obstetrical care but rather to illustrate that the chiropractor is an appropriate and necessary health care partner in the care of the pregnant woman.

When one rules out the use of drugs, surgery and most imaging modalities because they are often unsafe and inappropriate during pregnancy, it becomes clear that the chiropractor has an important role in the care of the pregnant woman. With conditions such as sciatica, headaches and the like being quite common during this period, I believe that chiropractic has much to offer and should be the first and most natural choice for the woman who is pregnant.

Education, intraprofessionally as well as interprofessionally is of paramount importance, and it is in this spirit that this book is written–to inform practitioners that chiropractic is safe, natural and efficacious for the pregnant woman. ■

JMF

Dedication

Special thanks to a woman who not only typed this manuscript many times over but who knew and understood what was contained within it...GERTRUDE DEVLIN. Her sudden death has left us with a great void. Her tremendous love for the chiropractic profession and her deep understanding of the scope and possibilities that chiropractic could offer to the world, and especially to children and pregnant women...Gertrude, we miss you and I dedicate this book to you and your family. ■

Acknowledgments

I would like to take this opportunity to thank the many people who made this book possible.

First of all I thank Dr. Maxine McMullen. Maxine and her wonderful work with children and pregnant women has inspired a generation of chiropractors. It is with immense gratitude that I thank her for sharing her great insight and wisdom with me and with the profession. For believing in me. Thank you Maxine!

To the International Chiropractors Association who took the bold step in bringing the care of children and pregnant women into the forefront of the profession and the public. To its officers who supported this work, — Dr. James Gregg, Dr. Gary Street, and Dr. Fred Barge, thank you! For his untiring effort to promote the work of the ICA thank you Ron Hendrickson. And to Molly Rangnath, the woman who continually pulls it all off, and who has fought so valiantly for the right of the chiropractor to see children and without whose work this book could never be, a thank you could never be enough.

To my editors in the field, Dr. Sharon Mellot, and Dr. Nancy Newbold, thank you.

To Debbie Gemborowski for her support and guidance in seeing this to fruition, thank you.

To my friends who support me always, Joe and Elaine Mercante, Dr. Jeff Garson, Dr. Dan de la Torre, Ann and Pat McEvily, Arthur Maggiola, Lydia Kanych, Marge Bais, Dr. Benita Gross, Dr. Ann Henderson, Dr. Mauro Marinelli, Teresa Goetz, Dr. Harry Lodge, Beverly and Richard Small, Janice and Eric Solomon, Dr. Kathy Reilly, Bob and Marjorie Mottola, Katharine and Dan Darst, Daine Paolillo, Chris Reggina, Mary Cullen, Irene Radzwillas, Tania Martin, Suzanne Devlin, Helene Fiorentino, Suzanne and Gary Golio — thank you!

To Janice Solomon for her wonderful Forward and her support and trust throughout the years.

To Margo Diesenhouse Esq. for her help and support, thank you.

To my second "Mom" Rose thank you.

To my patients who continually trusted me with their pregnant bodies.

To those who have worked in the office, Mary, Helen, Gert and Andy...thank you for your daily support and hard work.

To my Dad in heaven who gave me patience and the belief that anything is possible.

To my mom Audrey and my brother Jay: thank you for always being there for me. Your continued love and support is the best thing in the world for me! ■

Forward

I met Joan Fallon when I was pregnant with my first child. My body was very uncomfortable, and although I was not a stranger to chiropractic adjustments, I was quite hesitant to be adjusted during the pregnancy.

My first impression of Joan was warmth. Her casual manner made me feel at home, and when she spoke she was confident and knowledgeable. I looked about the office and noticed antiques standing beside modern equipment. I would learn, in time, that Joan's approach to chiropractic and its role in childbearing was a reflection of this first meeting; an eclectic blend of healing methods creating an effective approach to parturition.

Through two subsequent pregnancies I had Joan's skillful care guiding me through the months before and after birth. At times the adjustments dramatically improved the discomforts. Unlike the standard opinion of obstetrics, "Grin and bear it until the confinement is over," Joan had solid answers and practical solutions. The most dramatic problem I had was during my third pregnancy. I had a severe dislocation of my pubic bone which left my pelvis locked in a paralyzing position. With Joan's extensive knowledge of pregnancy and its effect on the body she was able to realign the bone and help me maintain stability of the pubic symphysis throughout the remainder of the pregnancy.

My labors went quickly and the births were smooth. I truly believe the proper alignment of my body helped me to release and open up to the powerful sensations of birth. The rapid anatomical and hormonal changes that occur after birth left me with headaches and a sore, aching body. The postpartum chiropractic adjustments were particularly helpful and I found Joan's commitment to healing and nurturing paid off when I felt my recoveries were complete.

As a childbirth educator I have taught many pregnant couples and observed their health care. Few seem satisfied with the care they receive unless it has more of the holistic qualities that Joan provides. My role as an educator is to share knowledge and help facilitate change. One way I achieve this is by helping couples view birth from a woman-centered, holistic model. The model resembles a wheel with the pregnant woman's desires and needs at the center. Each spoke of the wheel represents those who help create the birth she wants. Caregivers include all practitioners that provide quality care for the pregnant woman, midwife and/or obstetrician, childbirth educator, chiropractor, therapist, etc.

Chiropractors are essential to the model because the adjustments address the physical changes of pregnancy. The wheel turns smoothly when all "spokes" cooperate with the pregnant woman and with each other by respecting individual expertise. The chiropractor who has the added knowledge of the intricacies of pregnancy helps to create the positive energy that keeps the wheel perpetuating health.

My personal experiences have taught me to listen to my intuition and to what my body is telling me. Discomfort and pain affects all levels of the pregnant woman. The more nurtured and cared for the better the outcome. We were very pleased that Joan was able to attend our third child's birth. As years of work together first as patient/doctor, then as colleagues in the childbearing field, it was only natural that she share the joy of welcoming our daughter into this world. Our spiritual kinship toward a better, healthier birth made this birth a phenomenal experience.

Childbirth would enter a new dimension for women if they had the skillful assistance of a chiropractor at their birth. I feel fortunate to know a woman so dedicated to helping women through one of the most dramatic transitions in their life. This book is Joan's tribute to pregnant women, mothers and their babies. She has helped make this a better world by sharing this knowledge with others. This book is like a rare jewel, worth searching for and so priceless. Once you find it you will guard it carefully for many years to come.

Thank you Joan.

All my love,

Janice Solomon
Mahopac, NY
October, 1993

1 Reproductive Neuroanatomy

The female reproductive system is divided into two sections: the internal and the external genitalia. While considering the anatomical and physiological changes that occur during pregnancy, it is important to know the normal anatomy, especially the innervation of the female reproductive tract.

Pelvis

The word pelvis is derived from the Latin word meaning 'dish' and in many ways the pelvis resembles an upside down cup. The measurements and significance of differences in pelvic sizes and shapes will be covered elsewhere in this text, but now we will concern ourselves with the basic structures.

When one follows the movement of the fetus as it descends through the pelvis, the most important aspect is that of the shape of the various places in the pelvis. The top part of the pelvis (the inlet) has a distinctively different shape than that of the midcavity or of the outlet (Figure 1).

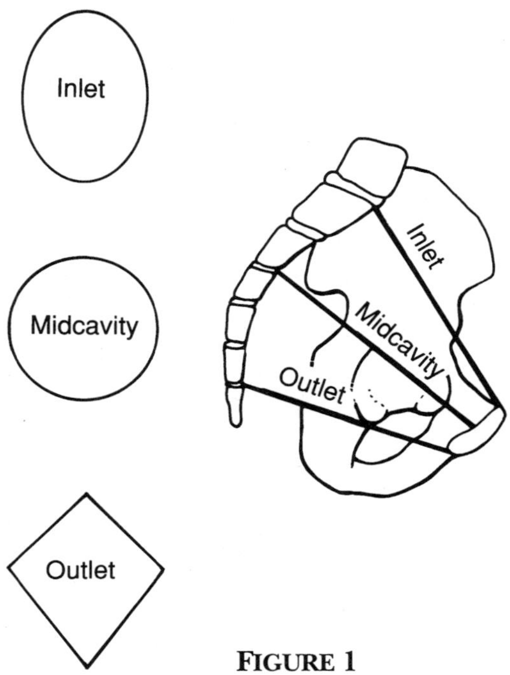

FIGURE 1

The lateral view of the pelvis shows the position of the uterus which is most often found in an anteverted position where the anterior wall of the vagina presses against the bladder. It is important to note the position of the rectum and to imagine the uterus enlarging during pregnancy and pressing against the rectum and the bladder (Figure 2).

The Perineum

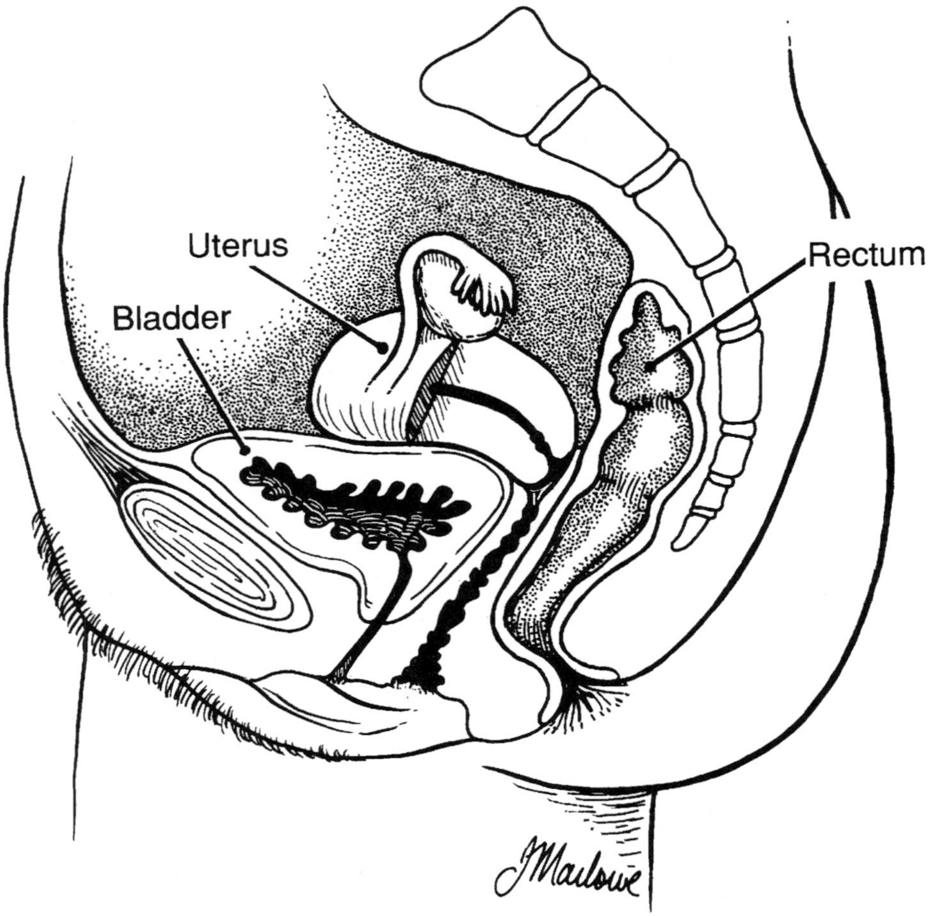

FIGURE 2

The perineum is the inferior boundary of the pelvis. It is bounded superiorly by the levator ani muscles and interiorly by the thighs (Figure 3). Anteriorly it is bounded by the symphysis pubis and posteriorly by the ishial tuberosities, the sacrotuberous ligaments and the coccyx (Figure 4). The muscles of the perineum divide it into two triangles, the urogenital triangle anteriorly and the anal triangle posteriorly.

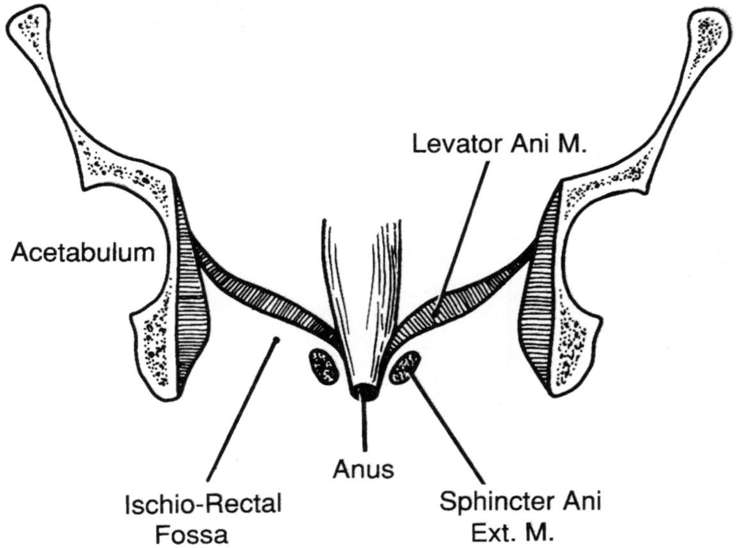

FIGURE 3

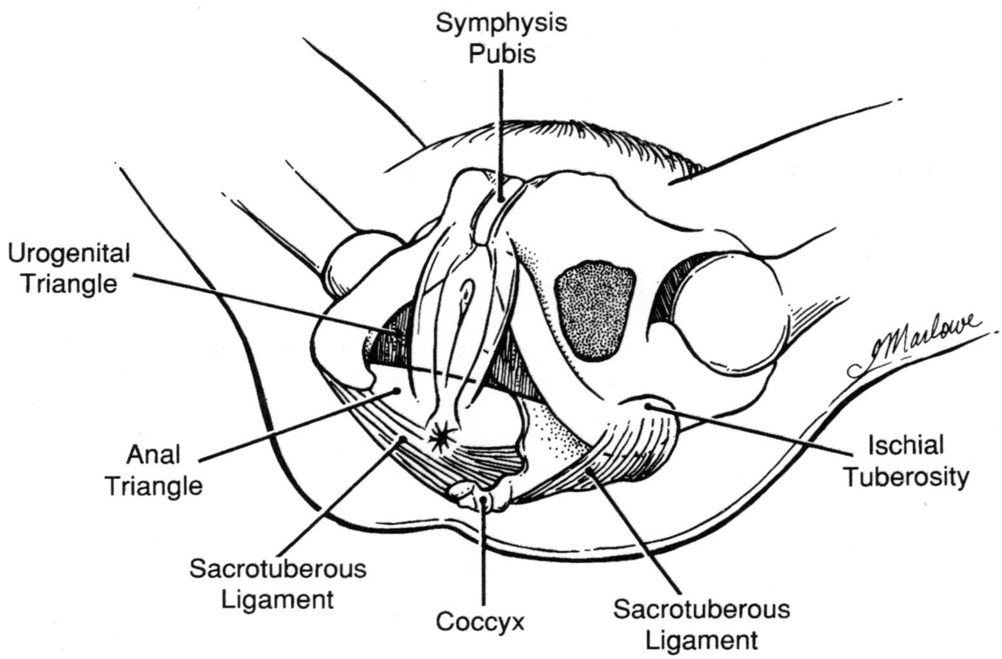

FIGURE 4

External Genitalia

The external genitalia is also known as the vulva. It includes the Bartholin's glands, clitoris, labia majora, labia minora, fourchette and the perineum. (Figure 5)

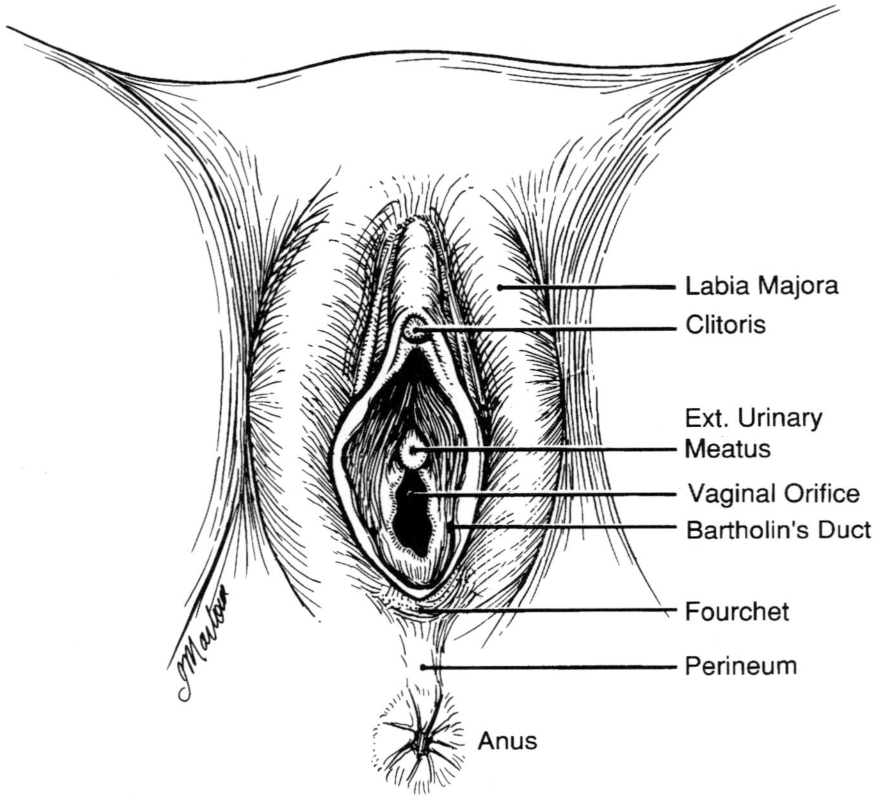

FIGURE 5

Vagina/Uterus

The vagina is the tube-like structure that reaches from the introitus to the fornices surrounding the cervix. It averages about 8 cm in length but varies with age, parity, and pre-post menopausal conditions.

The uterus is divided into three segments: the cervix, the isthmus and the body (Figure 6). The body is a pear-shaped organ lined with endometrium. There are four paired sets of uterine ligaments which attach to the uterus. These ligaments help to keep the uterus in place and as we will see later are affected by the physiological changes that occur during pregnancy. The transverse cervical ligaments are most important for support as compared to the other paired ligaments.

Fallopian tubes/ovaries

The fallopian tubes connect the uterus to the peritoneal cavity. The ovaries which contain the gamete material connect to the fallopian tubes which ultimately communicate with the uterus (Figure 6).

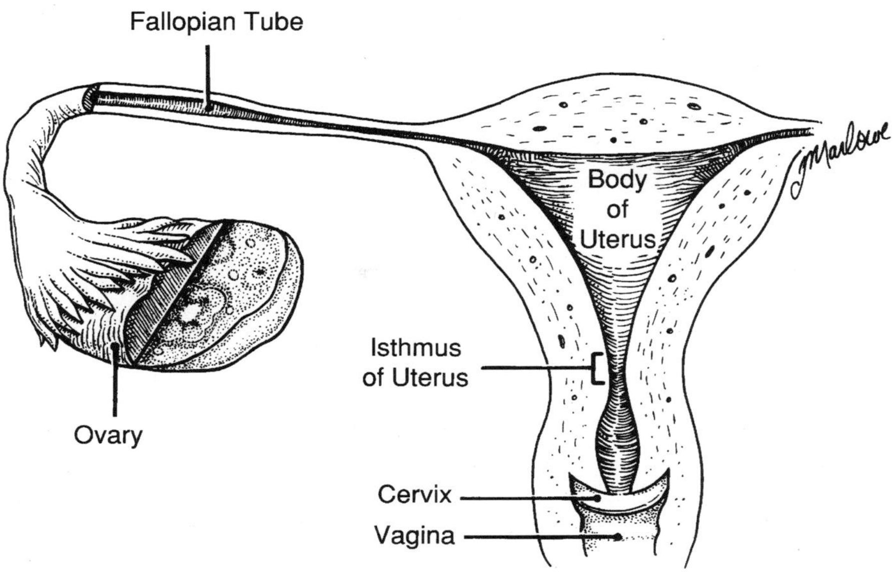

FIGURE 6

The nerve supply to the pelvic structures

In general, sympathetic innervation will cause muscular contraction and vasoconstriction. On the other hand, parasympathetic innervation will cause muscular relaxation and vasodilation, with the majority of autonomic innervation entering the pelvis by way of the superior hypogastric plexus. It is important to note that sympathetic innervation will cause the uterine muscle to relax. This has special significance during pregnancy.

The organs of the pelvis are innervated by both sympathetic and parasympathetic nerves. The sympathetic nerves originate from the lumbar sympathetic ganglia 1,2,3, and 4. They pass from the preaortic plexus down the uterovaginal plexus and the ovary (Figure 7). The sympathetic supply to the ovary which also corresponds to its visceral supply originates from T10 and T11. The uterus is innervated by visceral sensory nerves as well as autonomic fibers. Nerve cell bodies are not found in the uterus which originally led scientists to believe that the uterus was not at all under the control of the nervous system. Subsequent anatomical investigations however, revealed that nerve processes exist in all parts of the uterus with a large density found in the cervix and lower uterine segment. Fibers of the aortic

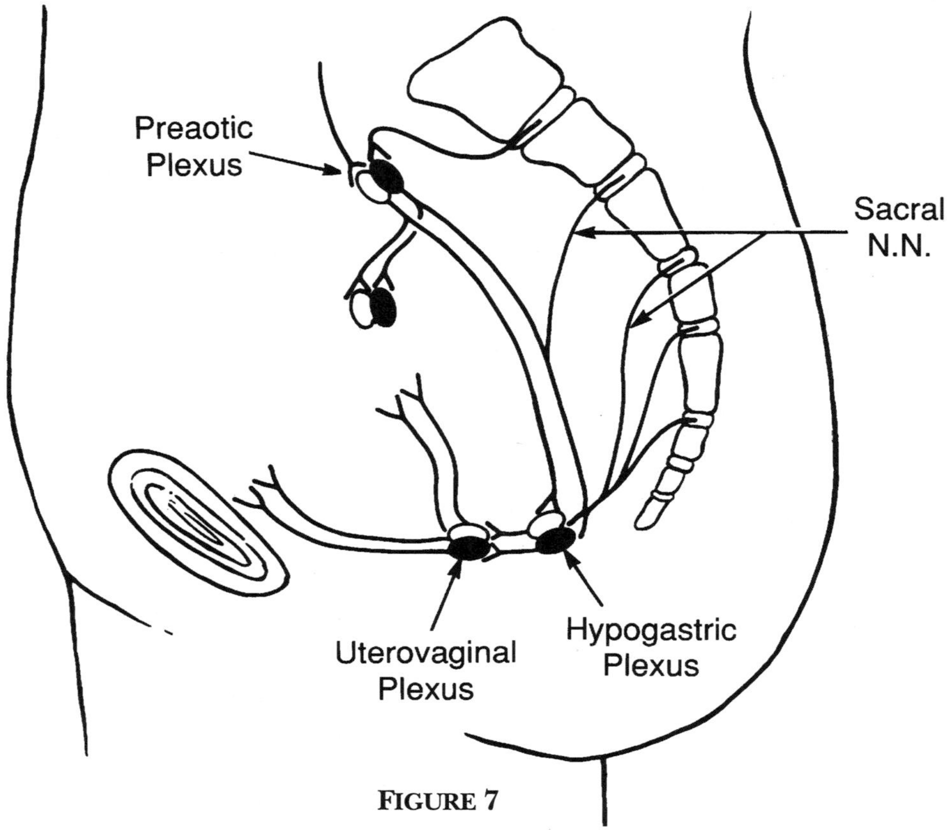

FIGURE 7

plexus form the superior hypogastric plexus and give rise to the sacral splanchnic nerves and the inferior hypogastric and ultimately the vaginal plexus. The sympathetic fibers come from the splanchnic group T6-L2, with the majority coming from T11, T12, L1. The sensory division enters the spinal cord at the doral roots of T11, T12, L1. Most all of the work that has been done in evidence of innervation of the pelvis and pelvic structures has been done prior to 1933 on extensive cadaver studies.

The upper vagina is virtually pain free, and there is little sensitivity to touch. The lower vaginal structures are most sensitive to pain and infection is often not perceived until it involves the vulva region. The labia and mons have extensive free nerve endings known as Merkel's discs. They are found in abundance in the lips and external genitalia of humans. The pudendal nerves innervate the intoitus for sensory perception and the motor fibers to the muscles of the pelvic floor. Thus a pudendal block will allow an episotomy to occur painlessly, but will not interfere with the course of the labor and delivery.

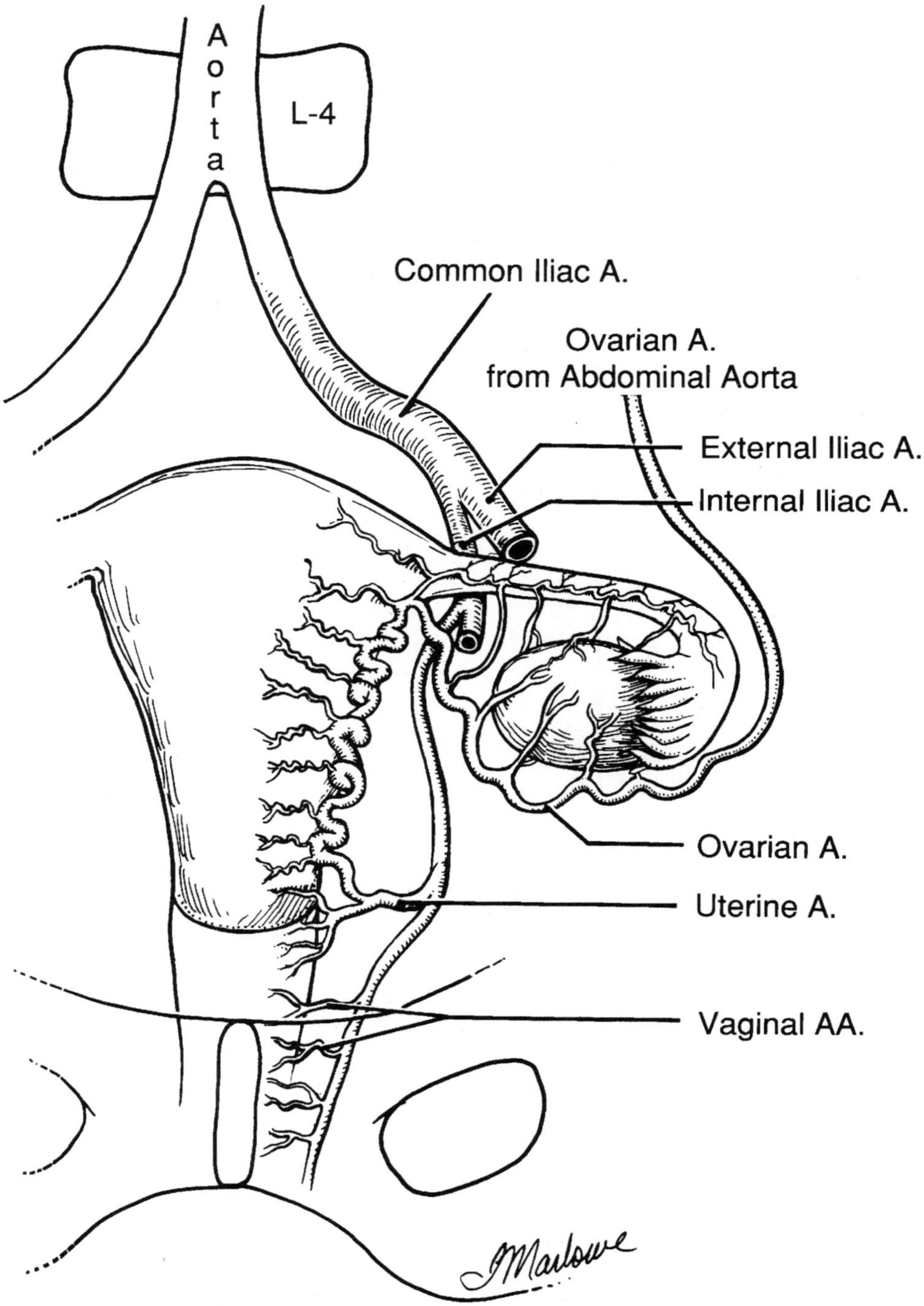

A
o
r
t
a
L-4
Common Iliac A.
Ovarian A.
from Abdominal Aorta
External Iliac A.
Internal Iliac A.
Ovarian A.
Uterine A.
Vaginal AA.

FIGURE 8

The vascular supply to the pelvic structures

The uterus and vagina receive their vascular supply from branches of the common iliac artery which give rise to the internal and external iliac arteries. The anterior branch of the internal iliac artery gives rise to the uterine, obturator and vaginal arteries. The ovaries receive their supply from the ovarian arteries which have their origin in the abdominal aorta and course their way to the ovaries by way of the posterior part of the pelvis over the pelvic brim. The ovarian arteries also supply the fallopian tubes and ultimately join the uterine arteries at that level (Figure 8).

Pain of childbirth

The pain of childbirth is associated with the dilatation of the cervix, uterine contraction and the stretching of the perineum. Sensory nerve input is carried from the uterus to the spinal cord by visceral afferent nerves which enter the spinal cord at T10, T11, T12, and L1. Pain fibers from the perineum travel to the spinal cord via somatic afferent nerves (pudendal nerve) and reach the spinal cord at the levels of S2, S3, and S4. These nerve impulses are carried to the brain via the spinothalamic tract.

Pelvic pain

One of the most common problems the chiropractor will encounter in the female patient is pelvic pain. It is important for the doctor to be able to differentiate the nature of the pelvic pain that presents in the office so that it is not misdiagnosed nor mistreated. Much of the pelvic pain which is treated gynecologically has its etiology in neuromuscular/subluxative origins.

The first step is to take a proper case history and perform a thorough neuromuscular skeletal examination. Many times the case history and physical examination will lead to the necessity of either a gynecological examination or further laboratory testing.

HISTORY

- type of discomfort and distribution and radiation of pain
- time and nature of onset
- duration of the pain
- relation to movement, urination, defecation, menstrual cycle, sleep, etc.
- other symptoms present

EXAMINATION

- regular examination: vitals, EENT, cardiovascular etc.
- reflexes, muscles testing
- orthopaedic testing
- careful palpation of the abdomen
- neurological testing
- spinal examination

The diagram on page 22 (Table 1) should serve as a guide to the differential diagnosis of pelvic pain. It is meant to serve as a guide and is in no way meant as a substitute for proper examinations.

Infertility & miscarriage as a result of subluxation

Miscarriage and infertility can result from any number of complex anatomical and physiological problems that the body possesses. Within each case there can be any number of variables which contribute to the problem. Regardless of the main etiology, one must consider the fact that subluxation can contribute and/or be a major factor. Dr. Julia Cochran of Louisville, Colorado designed a group of subluxation flow charts to use as a guide when seeing someone with infertility or chronic miscarriage. The charts on the following page are adapted from Dr. Cochran's work.

Sexual abuse

I have singled out this one aspect of possible pelvic pain etiology because it is so pervasive and so often overlooked. Recent statistics show that one in three women and one in five men are sexually abused. When the typical chiropractor sees 30 patients in a day, assuming a 50/50 ratio of men to women, the chiropractor may see on an average about 8 people a day who have been sexually abused.

The possibility of a history of sexual abuse should be especially considered when the patient presents with chronic pelvic pain or classical myofascitis which does not have its origin in a gynecological etiology and chiropractic adjustments appear to have little or no effect.

Cell memory of trauma is quite strong, and will often manifest itself in chronic pelvic pain. Sexual abuse victims, especially those who have suppressed their abuse will often experience a phenomena known as "flashback." When the flashbacks become very strong the cell memory of the trauma may be activated and the onset of pelvic pain may begin.

When the chiropractor encounters a patient who suffers pain of this nature, it is important to refer the patient for psychological treat-

CRANIAL SUBLUXATION

Pituitary Gland function

FSH | LH

Primary/Secondary Ovarian Function

Infertility | 1st Trimester Miscarriage

1ST CERVICAL VERTEBRA SUBLUXATION

Blood supply to Pituitary Gland | Sympathetic Nervous Function

(as above) | Organic Function

Infertility/Miscarriage

7TH CERVICAL VERTEBRA SUBLUXATION

Thyroid Gland Function

Anovulation

Infertility

9TH & 10TH THORACIC VERTEBRAE SUBLUXATION

Adrenal Gland Function

Decreased Ovulation | Adrenal Failure

Infertility

12TH THORACIC VERTEBRA SUBLUXATION

Fallopian Tube Function

Infertility | Ectopic Pregnancy

12TH THORACIC VERTEBRA SUBLUXATION

Ovarian Function
Maturation Release of Egg
Maintenance of Pregnancy

Uterine Function
Implantation Gestation of Fetus

Testicular Function
Maturation Release of Sperm

Penile Function
Erection Flow of Sperm

Infertility or Miscarriage

4TH LUMBAR VERTEBRA SUBLUXATION

Prostate Gland Function
Decreased Viability of Sperm
Infertility

SACRAL & COCCYGEAL SUBLUXATION

Function of Cervix

Menstrual Reflux
Endometriosis
Infertility

Cervical Incompetence
2nd Trimester Miscarriage

COLICKY	SUDDEN & UNREMITTING				GRADUAL & REMITTING			
	Fever & WBC		*No Fever*					
	VOMITING	NO VOMITING	EXACERBATED BY MOVEMENT	NOT EXACERBATED BY MOVEMENT	MUSCULO-SKELETAL	GI	OTHER	PSYCHO-LOGICAL
chronic cholecystitis chronic appendicitis intestinal malfunction food allergy subluxation	early acute appendicitis acute cholecystitis pyelonephritis bowel dysfuntion peritonitis	ruptured ovarian cyst ruptured ectopic pregnancy acute salpingitis parametritis pyelonephritis bowel obstruction acute bladder infection	torsion of ovarian cyst intraperitoneal irritation early appendicitis tumor subluxation	tumor degeneration of uterine myoma tumor bladder infection subluxation	congenital malformation tumor of soft tissue osteomyelitis ostecarthritis tumor subluxation	diverticulitis spastic colon	prolapsed uterus prolapsed bladder cystocele rectocele bladder infection	hysterical pregnancy childhood sexual abuse history of rape

TABLE 1

Differential Diagnosis of Pelvic Pain

ment. There are specialists who treat this condition exclusively, and who will understand that chiropractic care is a part of the multidisciplinary approach to this patient.

Anesthesia during birth

In recent years there is a trend towards natural childbirth with a decreased use of anesthetics and analgesics during birth. Anesthetics and analgesics can be administered either centrally (systemically) or locally. At this time locally administered drugs are the choice among young parents who choose to use medication during childbirth, due to the fact that systemic drugs most often cross the placental barrier and have an anesthetic/analgesic effect on the child which could reduce the heart rate or respiratory rate thereby possibly complicating the birth. ■

REFERENCES

Anatomy & Physiology

Austin CR: Fertilization. Englewood Cliffs, N.J., Prentice-Hall, 1965

Austin CR: Sperm maturation in the male and female genital tracts. In Metz CB,Monray A (eds): Biology of Fertilization, Volume 2, New York, Academic Press, 1985

Braude P, Bolton V, Moore S: Human gene expression first occurs between the four- and eight-cell stages of the preimplantation development. Nature, 332:459, 1988

Braunstein GD, Rasor JL, Engvall E, et.al.: Interrelationships of human chorionic gonadatropin, human placental lactogen and pregnancy-specific glycoprotein throughout normal human gestation. Am J Obstet Gynecol, 138:1205, 1980

Csapo AL, Pulkkinen MO: Indispensability of the human corpus luteum in the maintenance of early pregnancy luteectomy evidence. Obstet Gynecol Surv, 33:69, 1978

Eastman NJ, Hellman LM: Williams Obstetrics, 13th ed. New York, Appleton-Century-Crofts, 1966

Fallon JM: Orthopedic and neurological conditions of pregnancy, Multimedia Presentation, 1990

Fallon JM: The biomechanical and hormonal considerations of pregnancy as they relate to chiropractic care, Multimedia presentation 1989, 1993

Gill TJ III, Immunity and Pregnancy. CRC Crit Rev Immunol, 5:201, 1985

Grant JCB: An Atlas of the Human Body. 7th ed. Baltimore, Williams and Wilkins, 1978

Hearn JP: The embryo-maternal dialogue during early pregnancy in primates. J Reprod Fertil, 76:809, 1986

Hunziker RD, Wegmann TG, Placental immunoregulation. CRC Crit Rev Immunol, 6:245, 1987

Knobil E, Neill J (eds): The Physiology of Reproduction, New York, Raven Press, 1988

Lenton EA, Neal LM, Sulaiman R: Plasma concentrations of human chorionic gonadatropin from the time of implantation until the second week of pregnancy. Fertil Steril, 37:773, 1982

Ludwig H, Metzer H, The Human Female Reproductive Tract. A Scanning Electron Microscope Atlas, Heidelberg, Springer-Verlag, 1976

McMullen M: Assessing cervical subluxations in infants under six months of age. Articles on Pediatrics Vol I. International Review of Chiropractic, 1994

Moore KL: The Developing Human, 4th ed. Philadelphia, WB Saunders, 1988

Pauerstein CJ, Hodgson BJ, Kramen MA: The anatomy and physiology of the oviduct. Obstet Gynecol, Ann 3:317, 1974

Scott JR., DiSaia PJ, Hammond CB., Spellacy WN. Danforth's Obstetrics and Gynecology 6th ed. Philadelphia, J.B. Lippincott Company, 1990

Sholls HT, Orsini MW, Hitchins DJ: Estrogen synthesis and metabolism in the hamster blastocyst, uterus and liver near the time of implantation. J Steroid Biochemistry, 19:1153, 1983

Ulfelder H: Mechanism of pelvic support in women. Am J of Obstet Gynecol, 72:856, 1956

Wynn RM (ed) Cellular Biology of the Uterus, New York, Appleton-Century-Crofts, 1967

Neuromuscular Skeletal System

Adour KK: The bell tolls for decompression? New Eng J Med, 292:748, 1975

Aminoff MJ: Neurological disorders and pregnancy. Am J Obstet Gynecol, 132:325, 1978

Bell C: The Nervous System of the Human Body. London: Longman Rees, Orme, Brown, and Green, 1830

Berg G, Hammer M, Moller-Nielson J, et.al.: Low back pain during pregnancy. Obstetrics and Gynecology, 72:71

Berkwitz NJ and Lufkin NH: Toxic neuronitis of pregnancy: A clinicopathological report. Surgery, Gynecology and Obstetrics, 54:743, 1932

Benson RC, Inman VT: Brachialgia statica dysesthetica in pregnancy. Western Journal of Surgery, 64:115, 1956

Brown JT and McDougall A: Traumatic maternal birth palsy, Journal of Obstetrics and Gynecology of the British Empire, 64:431

Cole JT: Maternal obstetric paralysis, Am J Obstet Gynecol, 52:386

Ecker AD and Woltman HW: Meralgia parestetica: A report of one hundred and fifty cases, J Amer Med Assoc, 110: 1650, 1938

Eckman-Ordeberg G, Salgeback S, Ordeberg G: Carpal tunnel syndrome in pregnancy. A prospective study. Acta Obstet Gynecol Scand, 66:233, 1987

Fallon JM: Orthopedic and neurological conditions of pregnancy and chiropractic management of care, Articles on Pediatrics, International review of Chiropractic Vol II, 1994

Fallon JM: Orthopedic and neurological conditions of pregnancy, Multimedia Presentation, 1990, 1994

Fallon JM: The biomechanical and hormonal considerations of pregnancy as they relate to chiropractic care, Multimedia presentation 1989, 1993, 1994

Fisher AP, Hanna M: Transcutaneous nerve stimulation in meralgia parestetica of pregnancy, British J of Ob Gyn, 94:603, 1987

Font AT, Hankin RS: Pregnancy outcomes after now catastrophic maternal trauma during pregnancy. Obstet Gynecol, 35:912, 1970

Forster JB: Hydrocortisone and the carpal tunnel syndrome, Lancet, 1:456, 1960

Head HB,Welsh JS, Mussey E et.al.: Cyclic sciatica: Report of case with introduction of a new surgical sign. J Am Med Assoc, 180:521, 1962

Hamlin E, Lehman RAW: Carpal tunnel syndrome, New Engl J Med, 276:849, 1967

Jones MW, Berry K: Chronic relapsing polyneuritis associated with pregnancy, Transactions of the Obstetrical Society of London, 9:12, 1981

Ironside R: Neuritis complicating pregnancy, Proceedings of the Royal Society of Medicine, 32:588, 1939

King G, Ride LT: The relation of vitamin B1 deficiency to pregnancy toxemias. J of Obstet Gynecol of British Empire, 52:130, 1945

McMullen M: Assessing cervical subluxations in infants under six months of age. Articles on Pediatrics Vol I. International Review of Chiropractic, 1994

McMullen M: Handicapped children and chiropractic care (Part I & II). Articles on Pediatrics Vol 1. International Review of Chiropractic, 1994

O'Connell JEA: Lumbar Disc Protrusion in Pregnancy. J of Neurology, Neurosurgery and Psychiatry, 23:138, 1960

Prineas J: Peripheral nerve changes in thiamine-deficient rats. Archives of Neurology, 23:541, 1970

Sands RX: Backache of pregnancy: a method of treatment. Obstet Gynecol, 12:670, 1958

Sommerville BW: A study of migraines in pregnancy. Neurology, 22:824, 1972

Strauss MB, McDonald WJ: Polyneuritis of pregnancy: A dietary deficiency disorder. J Amer Med Assoc, 100:1320, 1933

Robinson JR, Pou JW: Bell's Palsy: A predisposition of pregnant women. Archives of Otolaryngology, 95:125,1972

Romberg MH:Diseases of the Nervous System Vol II, Sydenham Society, London, 1851

Urist MR: Obstetric fracture-dislocation of the pelvis: Report of a case with injury to the lumbosacral trunk and first sacral nerve roots. J of Am Med Assoc, 152:127, 1953

Anesthesia During Birth

Alpher MH: Toxicity of local anesthetics. New Eng J Med, 295:1432, 1976

Atrash HK, Koonin LM, Lawson HW, Franks AL, Smith JC: Maternal Mortality in the United States, 1979-1986. Obstet Gynecol, 76:1055, 1990

Friedman JM: Teratogen update: Anesthetic agents. Teratology, 37:69, 1988

Hellman K: Epidural anaesthesia in obstetrics. Canadian Anaesthetics Society, 12:398, 1965

Lamaze F: Painless childbirth: Psychoprophylactic Method. Chicago, Henry Regnery, 1970

Potts CR, Ullery JC: Maternal and fetal effects of obstetric anesthesia: Intravenous use of promethazine and meperidine. Am J Obstet Gynecol, 81:1253, 1961

Wagman IH, deJong RN, Prince DA: Effects of lidocaine on the central nervous system. Anesthes, 28:155, 1967

2 The Hormones of Pregnancy

The basis of all change that occurs during pregnancy is hormonal. Without the significant alterations of hormonal levels during pregnancy, there can be no viability of the fetus. The following are important hormonal levels of pregnancy.

Progesterone

Progesterone is produced by the corpus lutem of pregnancy during the first four weeks, and then subsequently is derived from the placenta. A maximum level of 250 mg/day is reached in the third trimester. The overall function of progesterone is to decrease the tonality and to relax the musculature. The following are its functions:

1. decreases smooth muscle tone
2. decreases vascular tone
3. increases temperature
4. increases fat storage
5. produces overbreathing/decreases pCO2
6. with estrogen enhances the development of the breasts

Estrogen

Estrogen peaks at 40 mg/day. It is produced early in pregnancy by the ovaries and later by the placenta. Estrogen is found in three forms. Estriol, estradiol, and estrone, of which 85% is found in the form of estriol which is produced by the placenta and fetal adrenal glands. The following are some of its functions:

1) produces a significant alteration in connective tissue increasing the mobility of the joint capsules, spinal segmental motor unit, and the pelvis
2) promotes the growth of the uterus and control of its function

3) with progesterone it helps to promote the development of the breasts
4) increases the water retention/conservation
5) reduces sodium excretion

The following hormones are important in pregnancy but play somewhat of a lesser role:

Cortisol

Cortisol is produced by the maternal adrenal glands early in pregnancy, and later by the placenta. It peaks at 25 mg/day. Its functions include increasing the normal blood sugar levels, as well as a possible role in the mediation of antibody activity.

Aldosterone

Aldosterone is produced by the maternal adrenal. It helps keep the sodium and water balance in the body.

HCG (Human Chorionic Gonadotropin)

HCG is produced approximately 10 days after fertilization. It is the hormone measured to determine the presence of a positive pregnancy. HCG, secreted by the growing trophoblast, sends a message back to the corpus luteum of the ovary to continue to produce high levels of estrogen and progesterone to preserve the pregnancy. Early nausea and vomiting have been theorized to be caused by high levels of HCG.

Prolactin

Prolactin, along with FSH (follicle stimulating hormone) and LH (leutinizing hormone)is produced by the anterior pituitary. Prolactin, while most commonly associated with lactation has another important function in maintaining the corpus luteum which in turn continues to promote the increased secretion of estrogen and progesterone.

Other hormones

There are many additional hormones which play important roles in the process of pregnancy, and they include: Relaxin which helps to soften the cervix and inhibits uterine motility; HCS (Human chorionic sommammotropin) has a function similar to prolactin, and the other gonadotropins FSH (follicle stimulating hormone), and LH (lutenizing hormone), which maintain the corpus luteum of pregnancy.

SYSTEMIC CHANGES ASSOCIATED WITH THE HORMONES OF PREGNANCY

During pregnancy each system of the body undergoes significant changes that can easily be observed by the chiropractor who cares for pregnant women. Each systemic change may reflect a problem that will be encountered by the chiropractor in the office, therefore a basic understanding of these changes is important.

Respiratory System

The changes that the respiratory system undergoes are due primarily to the hormonal effects of pregnancy and the physical increase in size of the uterus. The overall changes that occur with respect to the respiratory function of the lungs are reflected in Table 1.

INCREASE	DECREASE
tidal volume	respiratory reserve
respiratory rate	expiratory reserve
minute volume	residual volume
plasma ph	residual capacity
p O2	p CO2

TABLE 1

One of the most notable changes that occur is an increase in the circumference of the rib cage. This thoracic circumference increase is approximately 10 cm. It is reflected in a flattening of the costophrenic angle (Photos A & B). An increased movement of the diaphragm and an increase in the flaring of the ribs both contribute to this increase in the thoracic circumference. It is important to note that this change will produce the first sign of subluxation in the pregnant woman which may result in a condition known as intercostal neuralgia. (Figure 1) Pain in the mid-back region is a common complaint in the first trimester of pregnancy and is due to this alteration of the rib cage.

These changes are all representative of an overall increase in inspiration and expiration and take place in response to the increased needs of the fetus. (Table 2)

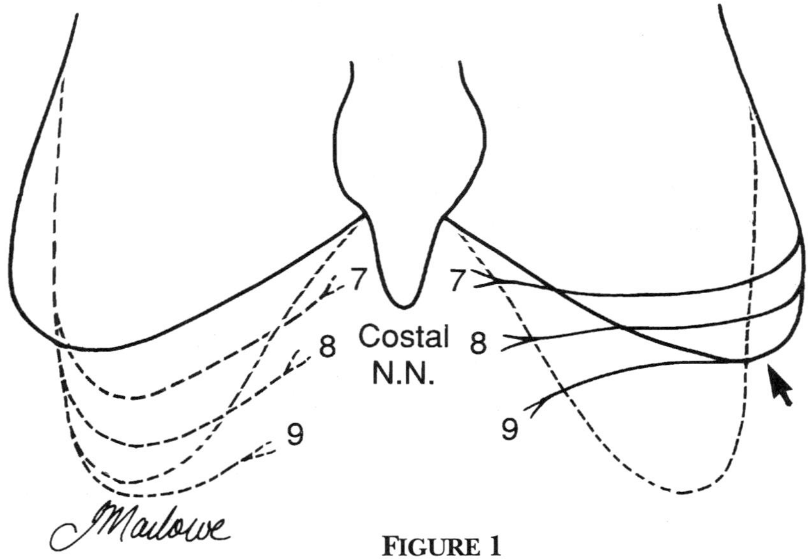

FIGURE 1

Picture A shows a non-pregnant woman. Note the breast overlay at the edge of the rib cage. Picture B shows a 24 week pregnant woman. Note the rib cage widening with the breast lying medial to the edge of the rib cage.

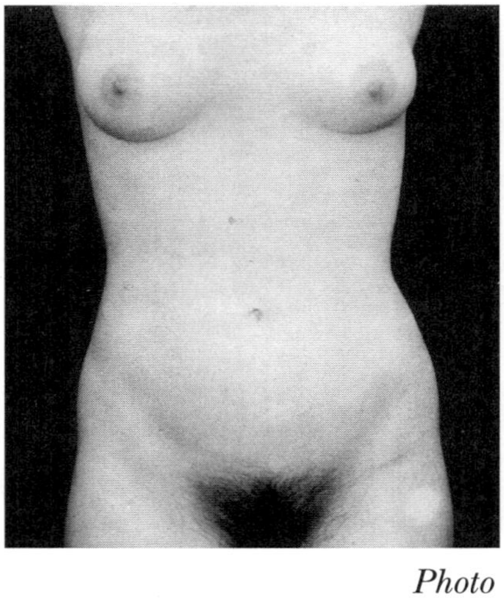

Photo A

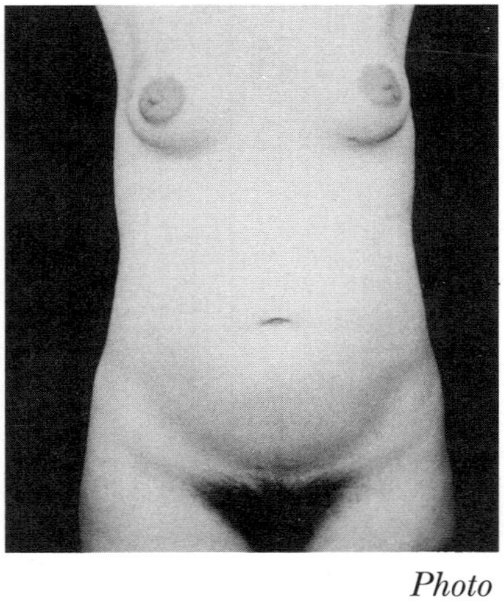

Photo B

INCREASED INSPIRATION	INCREASED EXPIRATION
↑ O2 uptake ⇩ ↑ pO2 ⇩ supply of O2 to the fetus	↑ CO2 Release ⇩ ↑ pCO2 ⇩ diffusion of CO2 to the mother

TABLE 2

Cardiovascular System

The changes that occur in the cardiovascular system are due to the greater demand for circulation to support the growing fetus and the hormonal changes which govern the overall expanded size of the vascular bed. During pregnancy the cardiovascular system increases in size by more than 50%. The demand for more circulation results in increased cardiac output, plasma volume, and number of vessels.

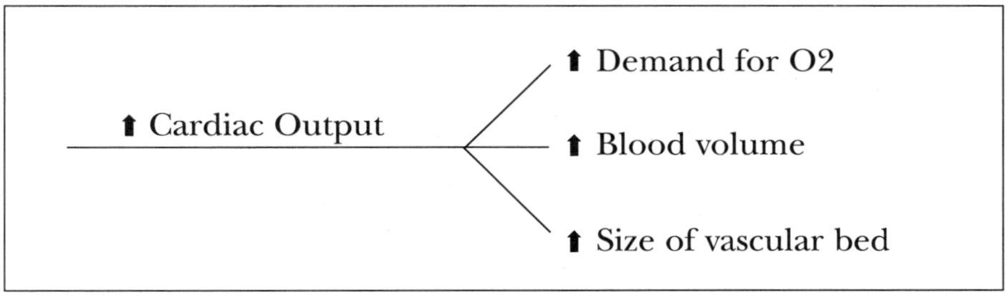

TABLE 3

If the cardiac output (CO) were allowed to increase without a concomitant change in the peripheral resistance and makeup of blood constitutents, the mother would become severely hypertensive which could lead to a tachycardia, MI, or most likely a CVA which may occur during labor. This increase in CO which increases the overall workload on the heart, is met by an equal reduction of workload on the heart which is accomplished mainly by a decrease in the peripheral resistance of the vascular bed (Table 4).

INCREASED CARDIAC WORK LOAD	DECREASED CARDIAC WORK LOAD
↑ blood volume	↑ peripheral vasodilation
↑ size of vascular bed	↑ # of red cells/ml plasma
	alteration of blood proteins

TABLE 4

While the total red cell volume increases approximately 18%, and the total plasma volume increases approximately 40-50%, there is an overall reduction in the hematocrit value (Hct). The hematocrit value is red cell volume/total plasma volume. This decrease in Hct is known as the *masked anemia of pregnancy* and is due solely to a hemodilution effect. This is a "normal" phenomena of pregnancy and should not be confused with other true anemic conditions of pregnancy.

Causes of Iron Deficiency Anemia During Pregnancy
Insufficient food intake
Morning sickness (hyperemesis gravidarum)
Diminished food absorption
-decreased gastric motility
-Vitamin C deficiency
Anemia preceding pregnancy
Multiple pregnancies
Insufficient time between pregnancies

Table 5

The three major anemia's of pregnancy are iron deficiency anemia, protein deficiency anemia, and folic acid deficiency anemia. Both protein deficiency and folic acid deficiency are a function of malnutrition or malabsorption. Iron deficiency anemia has many etiologies (Table 5).

One of the most commonly associated symptoms of pregnancy is the abnormal cravings that pregnant women often times experience. This is referred to as *The Pickle Pica of Pregnancy.* A pica is an abnormal craving for food usually associated with a nutritional deficiency, and in the case of the pregnant woman, is most often an iron deficiency. Pregnant women have been known to eat substances which range from pickles and ice cream to the margins of newspaper.

Gastrointestinal System

The changes that occur in the gastrointestinal system (GIS) are due to the hormonal effects of progesterone and estrogen, and result in an overall decrease in GI motility resulting in a severe slowing down of the entire system (Table 6).

Decreased GI Mobility	
Stomach ⇨	Nausea
Small Intestine ⇨	⬆ Absorption time
Large Intestine ⇨	⬆ H2O Absorption
	⬆ Constipation

Table 6

Water conservation and increased absorption time are the most important aspects of the GI changes during pregnancy. The growth of the fetus signals the maternal metabolism to increase appetite and to increase thirst. Usually a benign condition *hyperemesis gravidarum* (vomiting during pregnancy), also known as morning sickness, occurs during the first trimester. Occasionally it continues through the second and third trimester. When it is severe, this condition can lead to dehydration and possible liver damage. There are many theories why pregnant women suffer from morning sickness. Thought to be a function of the presence of high levels of HCG, it has been recently postulated that morning sickness is an evolutionary adaptive change to prevent the newly pregnant woman from ingesting foods that would be harmful to the developing fetus.

Renal System

The primary changes that occur in the renal system are actually secondary to the changes that occur in the cardiovascular system and the gastrointestinal system. There is a 30% - 50% increase in Glom-

FIGURE 2

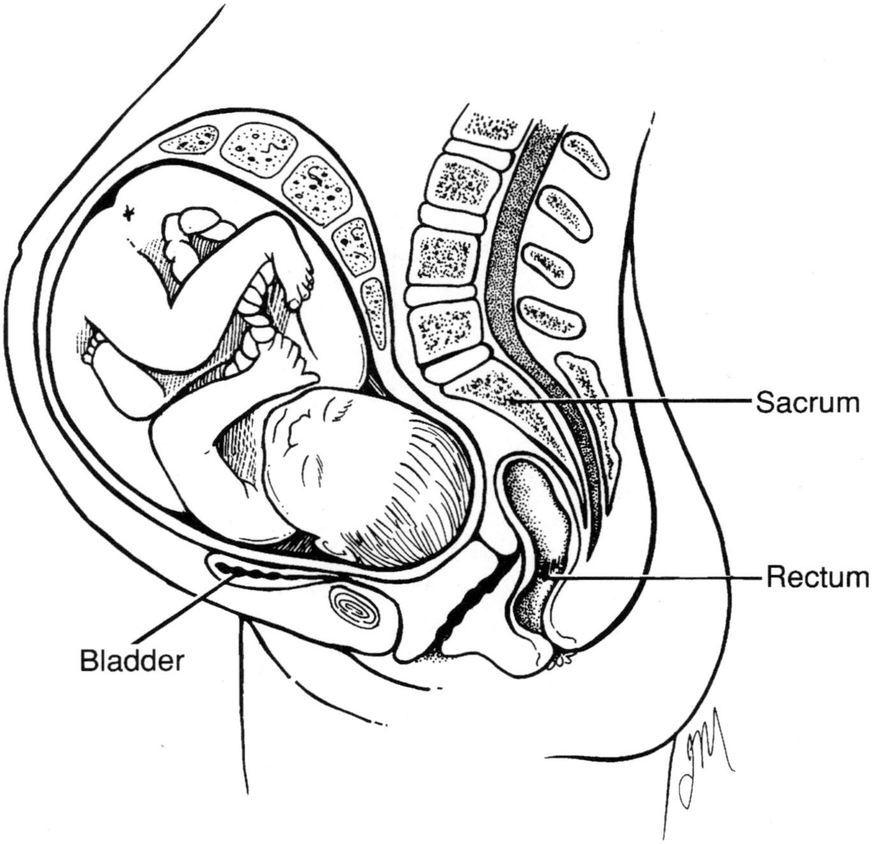

erular Filtration rate (GFR) due to an increase in cardiac output and increase in blood volume. Urine output however is decreased, due to an increase in tubular reabsorption.

While sleeping the pregnant woman will feel a need to urinate due to an increase in pressure on the great vessels in the supine position, which produces an increase in the GFR. There is also an increased frequency of urination. Early in pregnancy this is due to the enlargement of the uterus putting pressure on the bladder. Later in the pregnancy, the head of the baby puts pressure on the bladder stimulating the ejection reflex causing an increase frequency of urination.

Bladder and kidney infection is a problem that must be considered when treating the pregnant woman. Proper adjustments can minimize the possibility of infection by optimizing the innervation to the bladder. Progesterone which causes smooth muscle relaxation will cause the bladder to retain its fluid possibly longer than is optimum. Urine stagnation and incomplete emptying of the bladder increase the possiblity of infection. Proper innervation to the bladder will cause its proper emptying, thus minimizing the possibility of infection. ■

REFERENCES

Anatomy & Physiology

Austin CR: Fertilization. N.J., Prentice-Hall, Englewood Cliffs, 1965

Austin CR: Sperm maturation in the male and female genital tracts. In Metz CB, Monray A (eds): Biology of Fertilization, Volume 2, Academic Press, New York, 1985

Braude P, Bolton V, Moore S: Human gene expression first occurs between the four- and eight-cell stages of the preimplantation development. Nature, 332:459, 1988

Braunstein GD, Rasor JL, Engvall E, et.al.: Interrelationships of human chorionic gonadatropin, human placental lactogen and pregnancy-specific glycoprotein throughout normal human gestation. Am J Obstet Gynecol, 138:1205, 1980

Csapo AL, Pulkkinen MO: Indispensability of the human corpus luteum in the maintenance of early pregnancy luteectomy evidence. Obstet Gynecol Surv, 33:69, 1978

Eastman NJ, Hellman LM: Williams Obstetrics, 13th ed. Appleton-Century-Crofts, New York, 1966

Fallon JM: Orthopedic and neurological conditions of pregnancy, Multimedia Presentation, 1990

Fallon JM: The biomechanical and hormonal considerations of pregnancy as they relate to chiropractic care, Multimedia presentation 1989, 1993

Gill TJ III, Immunity and Pregnancy. CRC Crit Rev Immunol, 5:201, 1985

Grant JCB: An atlas of the Human Body. 7th ed. Williams and Wilkins, Baltimore, 1978

Hearn JP: The embryo-maternal dialogue during early pregnancy in primates. J Reprod Fertil, 76:809, 1986

Hunziker RD, Wegmann TG, Placental immunoregulation. CRC Crit Rev Immunol 6:245, 1987

Knobil E, Neill J (eds): The physiology of reproduction, Raven Press, New York, 1988

Lenton EA, Neal LM, Sulaiman R: Plasma concentrations of human chorionic gonadatropin from the time of implantation until the second week of pregnancy. Fertil Steril, 37:773, 1982

Ludwig H, Metzer H, The human female reproductive tract. A Scanning Electron Microscope Atlas, Springer-Verlag, Heidelberg, 1976

McMullen M: Assessing cervical subluxations in infants under six months of age. Articles on Pediatrics Vol I. International Review of Chiropractic, 1994

Moore KL: The Developing Human, 4th ed. Philadelphia, WB Saunders, 1988

Pauerstein CJ, Hodgson BJ, Kramen MA: The anatomy and physiology of the oviduct. Obstet Gynecol Ann, 3:317, 1974

Scott JR, DiSaia PJ, Hammond CB, Spellacy WN. Danforth's Obstetrics and Gynecology 6th ed. J.B. Lippincott Company, Philadelphia, 1990

Sholls HT, Orsini MW, Hitchins DJ: Estrogen synthesis and metabolism in the hamster blastocyst, uterus and liver near the time of implantation. J Steroid Biochemistry, 19:1153, 1983

Ulfelder H: Mechanism of pelvic support in women. Am J of Obstet Gynecol, 72:856, 1956

Wynn RM(ed) Cellular Biology of the Uterus, Appleton-Century-Crofts, New York, 1967

Hormones of Pregnancy

Baird DT: Preface. In Baird DT, Michie EA (eds.): Mechanisms of Menstrual Bleeding. Raven Press, New York, 1985

Bradbury JT, Brown WE, Guay LA: Maintenance of the corpus luteum and physiological action of progesterone. Recent Prog Horm Res, 5:151, 1950

Braunstein GD, Rasor JL, Engvall E, et.al.: Interrelationships of human chorionic gonadatropin, human placental lactogen and pregnancy-specific glycoprotein throughout normal human gestation. Am J Obstet Gynecol, 138:1205, 1980

Cassmer O: Hormone production of the isolated human placenta. Acta Endocrinol, 32 (suppl):45, 1959

Csapo AL, Pulkkinen MO: Indispensability of the human corpus luteum in the maintenance of early pregnancy luteectomy evidence. Obstet Gynecol Surv, 33:69, 1978

Eastman NJ, Hellman LM: Williams Obstetrics, 13th ed. Appleton-Century-Crofts, New York, 1966

Fallon JM: Orthopedic and neurological conditions of pregnancy, Multimedia Presentation, 1990,1994

Fallon JM: The biomechanical and hormonal considerations of pregnancy as they relate to chiropractic care, Multimedia presentation 1989, 1993,1994

Gill TJ III, Immunity and Pregnancy. CRC Crit Rev Immunol, 5:201, 1985

Hearn JP: The embryo-maternal dialogue during early pregnancy in primates. J Reprod Fertil, 76:809,1986

Hunziker RD, Wegmann TG, Placental immunoregulation. CRC Crit Rev Immunol, 6:245 1987

Khodr GS, Siler-Khodr TM: Placental lutenizing hormone-releasing factor and its synthesis. Science, 207:315,1980

Knobil E, Neill J (eds): The Physiology of Reproduction, Raven Press, New York, 1988

Lenton EA, Neal LM, Sulaiman R: Plasma concentrations of human chorionic gonadatropin from the time of implantation until the second week of pregnancy. Fertil Steril, 37:773, 1982

Potter EL, Craig JM: Pathology of the fetus and infant. Year Book, Chicago, 1975

Smout CFV, Jacoby F, Lillie EW: Gynecological and Obstetrical Anatomy. Williams and Wilkins, Baltimore, 1969

Nutrition

Begner L, Susser MW: Low birth weight and prenatal nutrition: An interpretive review. Pediatrics, 46:946, 1970

Fahey PJ, Boltri JM, Mark JS: Key issues on nutrition. From conception through infancy. Postgrad Med, 81:301, 1987

Hemminti E, Stanfield B: Routine administration of iron and vitamins during pregnancy: Review of controlled clinical trials. Br. J Obstet Gynecol, 85:404, 1978

Jarnfelt-Samisoe A: Nausea and vomiting in pregnancy. A review. Obstet Gynecol Surv, 42: 422, 1987

National Research Council: Alternative Dietary Practices and Nutritional Abuses during Pregnancy. National Academy of Sciences, Washington D.C. 1982

Piconce TA, Allen LH, Olsen PN, Fern MF: Pregnancy outcome in North American women. Ill effects of direct cigarette smoking, stress, and weight gain on placentas and on neonatal physical and behavioral characteristics. Am J Clin Nutr, 36:1214,1982

Weight Gain

Abrams BF, Lans RK: Prepregnancy weight, weight gain and birth weight. Am J Obstet Gynecol, 154:503, 1986

Gormician A, Valentine L, Satter E: Relationship of maternal weight gain, prepregnancy weight and infant birth weight. J Am Diet Assoc, 77:662, 1980

Systemic Changes During Pregnancy

Anderson LL: Regulation of relaxin secretion and its role in pregnancy. Adv Exp Med Biol, 219:421, 1987

Baird JD: Some aspects of the metabolic and hormonal adaptation to pregnancy. Acta Endocrinol, (suppl) (Copenh) 277:11, 1986

Brody SA, Ueland K (eds): Endocrine Disorders in Pregnancy, Appleton & Lange, Norwalk CT, 1989

Chesley LC, Sibai BM: Blood pressure in the midtrimester and future pre-eclampsia. Am J Obstet Gynecol, 157:1258, 1987

Davison JM: Kidney function in pregnant women. Am J Kidney Dis, 9:265, 1987

DeSwiet M: The respiratory system. In Hytten FE, Chamberlain G (eds): Clinical Physiology in Obstetrics, 2nd ed. Blackwell, Oxford, 1991

Douvas SG, Meeks GR, Phillips JC, et.al.: Liver disease in pregnancy. Obstet Gynecol Surv, 38:531, 1983

Easterling TR, Schumucker BC, Benedetti TJ: The haemodynamic effects of orthostatic stress during pregnancy. Obstet Gynecol, 72:550, 1988

Fallon JM: Orthopedic and neurological conditions of pregnancy, Multimedia Presentation, 1990

Fallon JM: The biomechanical and hormonal considerations of pregnancy as they relate to chiropractic care, Multimedia presentation 1989, 1993

Gant NF, Whalley PJ, Everett RB, et.al.: Control of vascular reactivity in pregnancy. Am J Kidney Disease, 9:303, 1987

Grant JCB: An Atlas of the Human Body. 7th ed. Williams and Wilkins, Baltimore, 1978

Klein EA: Urologic problems in pregnancy: A review. Obstet Gyecol Surv, 39:605, 1984

Lind T: Metabolic changes in pregnancy relevant to diabetes mellitus. Postgrad Med J, 55:353, 1979

Macfie AG, Magides AP, et. al.: Gastric emptying in pregnancy. Br J Anaesth, 67:54, 1991

Metcalfe J, McAnulty JH, Ueland K: Burwell and Metcalfe's Heart Disease in Pregnancy: Physiology and Management. Little, Brown, Boston, 1986

Milne JS, Howie AD, Pack AI: Dyspnoea during normal pregnancy. Br. J Obstet Gynecol, 85:260, 1978

Pritchard JA, Scott DE: Iron stores of normal adults and their replenishment with oral iron therapy. J Am Med Assoc, 190:897, 1964

Smout CFV, Jacoby F, Lillie EW: Gynecological and Obstetrical Anatomy. Williams and Wilkins, Baltimore, 1969

3 Prenatal Care

One of the most important aspects of pregnancy is prenatal care which includes chiropractic care. We will see in other parts of this text that chiropractic care is actually an integral part of the prenatal and postpartum care of the pregnant woman. Prenatal care is defined as the care and assessment of the growing fetus and the mother. The recent emphasis on prenatal care is the result of studies which show that women who have good prenatal care reduce the overall infant mortality and morbidity. Chiropractic care is essential to the pregnant woman for both her well-being and that of the growing and developing baby.

Once the initial exam is performed and a positive diagnosis of the pregnancy is confirmed, testing and measuring of the mother and the growing fetus is the next step in the practitioner's management of care program.

Diagnosis of pregnancy

At one time the diagnosis of pregnancy was strictly the domain of the obstetrician. Many of the old-time movies had scenes where the doctor came out of his examination room and informed the woman that she was "going to have a baby." The arena for that has changed to the home where women who miss their periods can do a home pregnancy test to determine a positive pregnancy.

The determination of pregnancy is broken into three categories: positive, probable, and presumptive. A positive determination is made by either visualizing the fetus, detecting a heartbeat or the perception of fetal movements. With the development of the Doppler fetascope, the detection of the heartbeat can be done significantly earlier (10-12 weeks). Echocardiography can detect the presence of a fetal heartbeat at 5-6 weeks.

Some of the presumptive signs of pregnancy include cessation of the menses, amenorrhea, breast enlargement, and changes in skin pigmentation. Signs such as Hegar's sign, which is the softening of the cervix upon bimanual examination, and internal ballotment which is the detectable movement of the fetus and audible tap heard when pressure is applied upwards to the cervix, are still the main signs used by the obstetrician.

At 18 weeks or thereabout the pregnant woman can begin to feel the life within. This is known as *quickening*. At approximately 15-16 weeks the enlargement of the abdomen is perceptible and the fundal height (top) of the uterus grows until 38 weeks at which time the fetus begins its descent into the lower segment of the cervix. This is known as *lightening*.

The following are signs of pregnancy and the gestational order in which they appear:

4 weeks - amenorrhea/morning sickness
6 weeks - breast changes/Doppler fetal heart beat
7 weeks - palpatory uterine changes
8 weeks - Hegar's sign
9 weeks - uterus is palpatory abdominally
13 weeks - ballotment
16 weeks - quickening in a multiparous/ abdominal enlargement
18 weeks - quickening in the primiparous
20 weeks - palpatory uterine contractions/ palpatory fetal movements
24 weeks - fetal heart audible with fetascope
26 weeks - palpatory fetal parts

Initial Visit

- determination of positive pregnancy
- history/physical exam
- laboratory testing CBS, SMAC, Blood type, Rh, Rubella, Hep B, HIV, Chlamydia
- discuss birth plan
- breast examination

Skin changes in pregnancy

Very often the pregnant woman wears the signs of pregnancy on the outside. She has on her face what is known as the mask of pregnancy or *cloasma*. This is the increase in pigmentation which occurs not only in the face but in the areolar area and external genitalia. In addition she may have an increased line of pigmentation which stretches from the symphysis pubis to the umbilicus. In addition, stretch mark–like streaks may appear on the abdomen, buttocks, breasts and thighs known as striae gravidarum. Often these marks, unlike others, do not disappear.

The initial visit to the obstetrician/midwife is an extensive visit consisting of a thorough physical examination, and a consultation. Baseline blood and urine testing is usually performed as well as a risk assessment. When the pregnant woman enters the chiropractor's office a specific examination should be performed. Unlike the obstetrician or midwife, the chiropractor may not have the benefit of early intervention, and the pregnant woman may present in the office days before delivery. If the pregnant woman is unfamiliar with the benefits of chiropractic care during this time, she will most likely present with back pain that may or may not be debilitating. The etiology of that pain must first be differentially diagnosed before treatment. In Chapter 1 we examined the differential diagnosis of pelvic pain in the non pregnant woman. In the pregnant woman this is not as simple and care must be given to this process.

Some abnormal conditions which may present with pelvic/abdominal/and or back pain during pregnancy are:

1) urinary calculus
   S/S • acute pain which radiates into the groin
   • possible hematuria

2) ovarian cyst
   S/S • torsion of an ovarian cyst may cause vomiting and tenderness of the abdomen

3) bowel obstruction
   S/S • adhesive bands are formed as uterus grows and pushes into the abdomen
   • occasionally a volvulus can occur

4) appendicitis
   S/S • point of maximum tenderness (PMT) is higher in pregnancy
   • the usual level of inflammation and irritation is reduced due to the high hormonal levels

5) degenerating fibroids
   S/S • pain, vomiting, and tenderness of the lower abdomen

6) perforation of a peptic ulcer
   S/S • rare due to the high hormone levels, especially during the third trimester

Fundal Height – The following illustration (Figure 1) depicts the classical fundal heights of the uterus as it progresses through pregnancy. It is important to note that at about 38-40 weeks the fundal height drops. This drop is known as lightening. This is most noticeable in the primagravida.

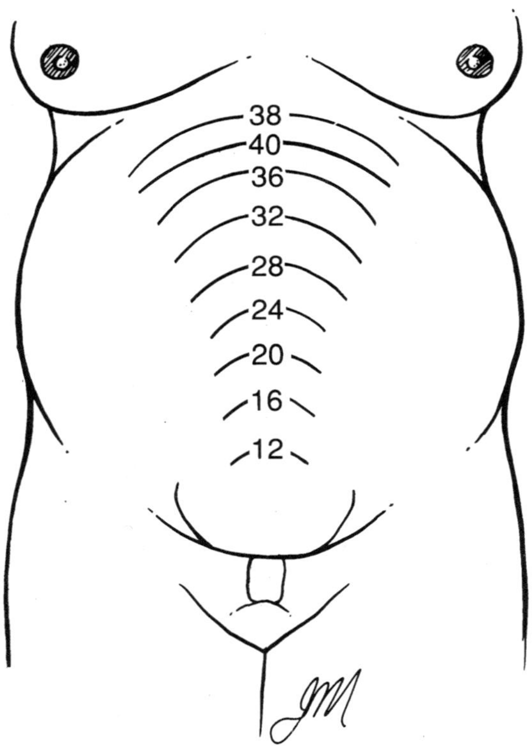

FIGURE 1

VAGINAL BLEEDING DURING PREGNANCY

Very often the pregnant woman will experience vaginal bleeding during the course of her pregnancy. It is important to differentiate the nature of the bleeding and to understand its relationship to possible problems during the pregnancy. The following are some of the types of bleeding that may be experienced during pregnancy:

Ectopic Pregnancy

An ectopic pregnancy is defined as a pregnancy where the products of conception are developing outside the uterus. The most common site of ectopic pregnancy is the fallopian tube. In the tube there is little or no submucosa and there is no decidual reaction so the muscle is easily invaded by the trophoblast. Because of the small amount of musculature in the tube it will not expand but rather rupture as the trophoblast begins to grow.

Some of the predisposing factors which increase the possibility of an ectopic pregnancy are:

1) IUD use
2) prior tubal or pelvic infection
3) congenital abnormalities of the tube

The signs and symptoms (s/s) of an ectopic pregnancy may include:

- pain/uterine colic
- stabbing or cramp-like pain in the lower abdomen
- referred pain to the shoulder if the phrenic nerve is involved
- vaginal bleeding

The vaginal bleeding may be extensive and occurs as the death of the ovum occurs and there are estrogen withdrawal symptoms. There is however no vaginal bleeding in 25% of ectopic pregnancies. Very often there is an acute internal hemorrhage which may cause shock. Acute internal blood loss is the most dramatic and dangerous complication of an ectopic pregnancy.

During a pelvic examination there is most often extreme pain over the gravid tube. There may also be an extreme peritoneal irritation with muscle guarding, fever and an increased frequency of micturition.

Abortion – A natural abortion (miscarriage) may result in abnormal bleeding. Any sign of bleeding during pregnancy should be brought immediately to the attention of the obstetrician/midwife.

Ante-partum Hemorrhage – Occurs after 28 weeks and may be caused by a placenta praevia or an abruptio placenta. An abruptio placenta is a placenta which spontaneously separates from the wall of the uterus. Placenta praevia is an abnormally situated placenta which is being irritated by the positioning of the fetus.

Intrapartum Hemorrhage – Hemorrhage that occurs during the birth process. It may occur as a result of an abruptio placenta, a placenta praevia, a vasa praevia, or excessive blood flow at the onset of labor.

Post-Partum Hemorrhage – Any type of trauma to the vagina, perineum, or cervix may cause hemorrhage after the birth. A retained cotyledon may also present abnormal bleeding after birth.

Other Causes –

- Cervical carcinoma
- Varicosities

- Cervical erosion
- Cervical polyps
- Hemorrhoids
- Urinary tract infection

Toxemia of pregnancy

Classical toxemia is known as eclampsia, and the true disease process begins before it becomes full eclampsia. It is known as pre-eclampsia. This is a disease of the second half of pregnancy and may have no marked signs or symptoms. The cardinal signs of pre-eclampsia are:

1) Hypertension: always present
2) Proteinuria: always present
3) Excessive edema: sometimes present

The etiology of toxemia is unknown and has eluded complete understanding for as long as women have been giving birth. At present the widely accepted theory is that poor nutrition is the root of toxemic changes, since poor nutrition is synonymous with inadequate absorption of nutrients. Other possible causes may be:

- Intravascular fibrin deposition
- Failure of the immune response
- Excessive uterine distension
- Water and salt retention

In addition to the three cardinal changes in a well developed pre-eclampsia, there are two additional changes that occur:

4) Blood coagulation changes - increased activation of the blood clotting system
5) Renal changes - a reduction of renal function
   - an increase in uric acid, plasma urea and creatinine

When pre-eclampsia develops into eclampsia the following may develop:

1) epilepsy
2) sub-arachnoid/cerebral hemorrhage
3) preexisting brain tumors may fulminate
4) uremia
5) liver failure
6) placental necrosis
7) glomerular and tubular necrosis

Ultrasound in pregnancy

The imaging test of choice in pregnancy is ultrasound. Performed routinely at least once during the pregnancy, its efficacy has been debated for many years both in the medical and non-medical fields.

It is easiest to think of ultrasound as sound produced energy (Figure 2). Any energy that is placed into a living organism will produce some type of change. Whether that change is helpful or deleterious, or whether that change is less important than the information gleaned from the test are the issues that must be examined when giving advice about ultrasound.

SOUND WAVES ⇨ ENERGY ⇨ CHANGE

The frequency of ultrasound is 3.5 5 mHz and its intensity is measured in watts or mwatts/sq cm of tissues exposed. A sound wave is capable of making a change that is either thermal, vibrational, or mechanical in nature. During the first trimester the cells are rapidly dividing and are undifferentiated. When the fetus reaches the third trimester the cells become highly differentiated and continue to divide. Change that occurs in differentiating tissue can potentially cause a deleterious mutation in a cell.

There are several uses of ultrasound which may be important and must not be overlooked. These include:

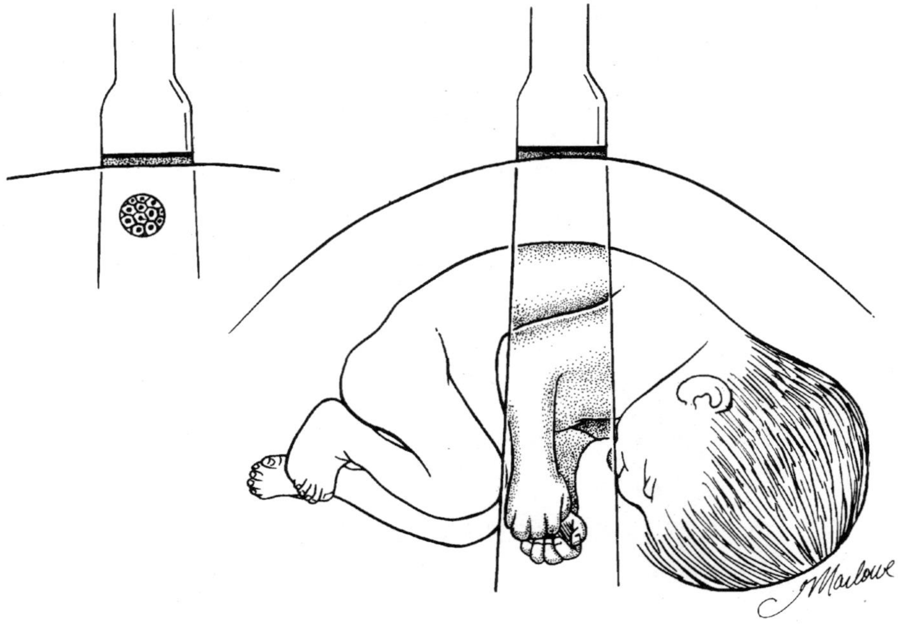

FIGURE 2

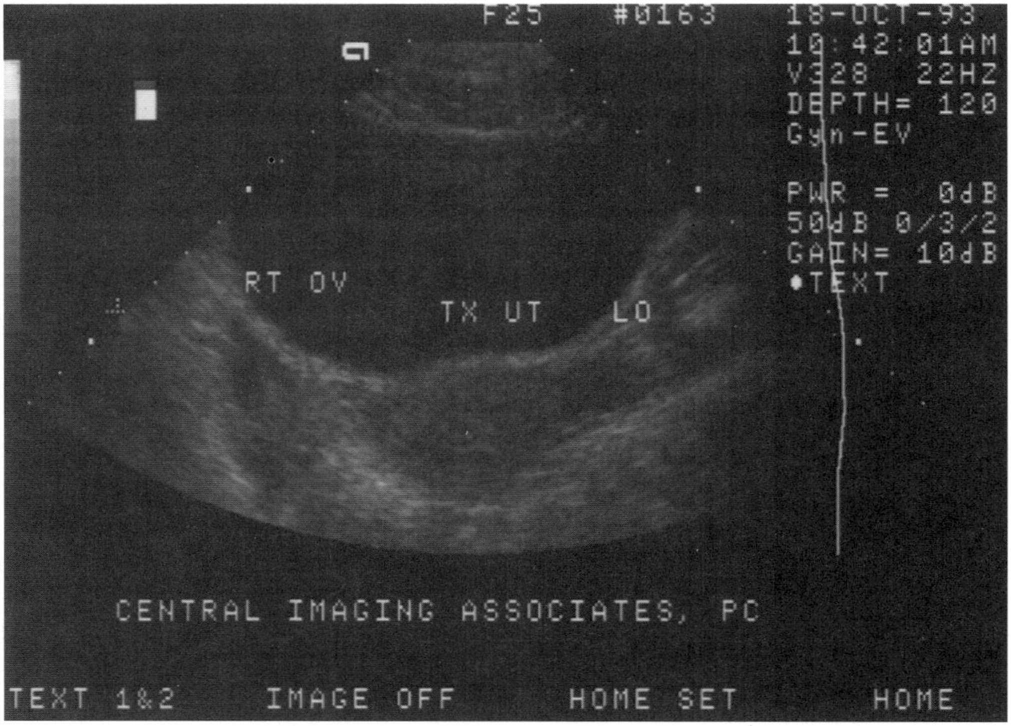

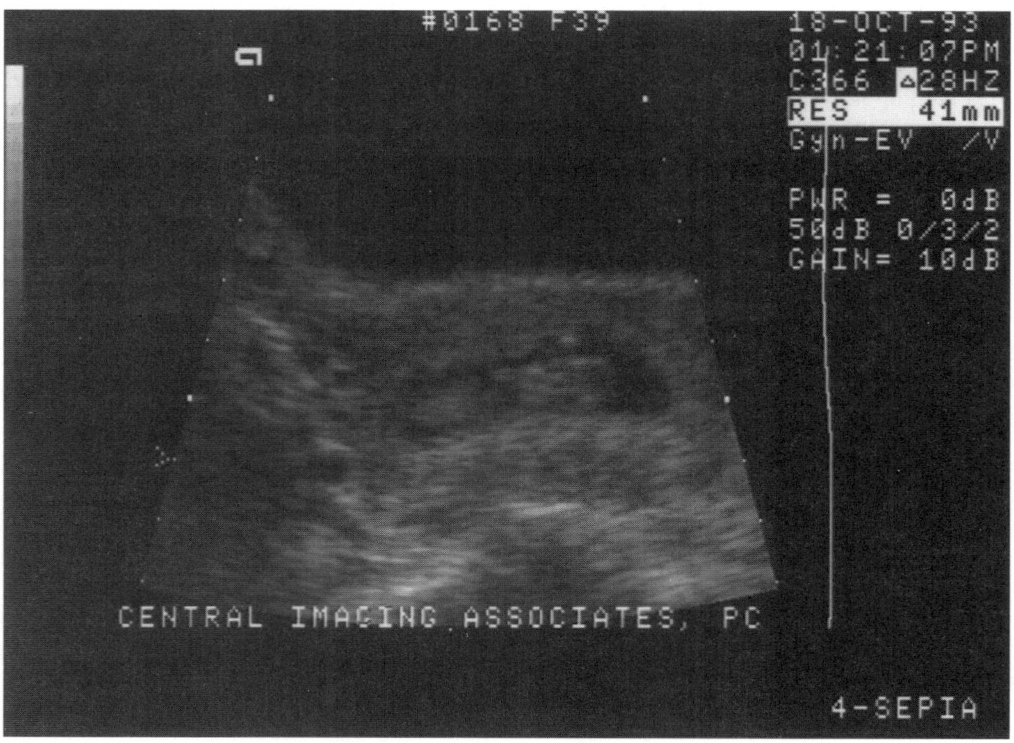

ULTRASOUND IMAGING

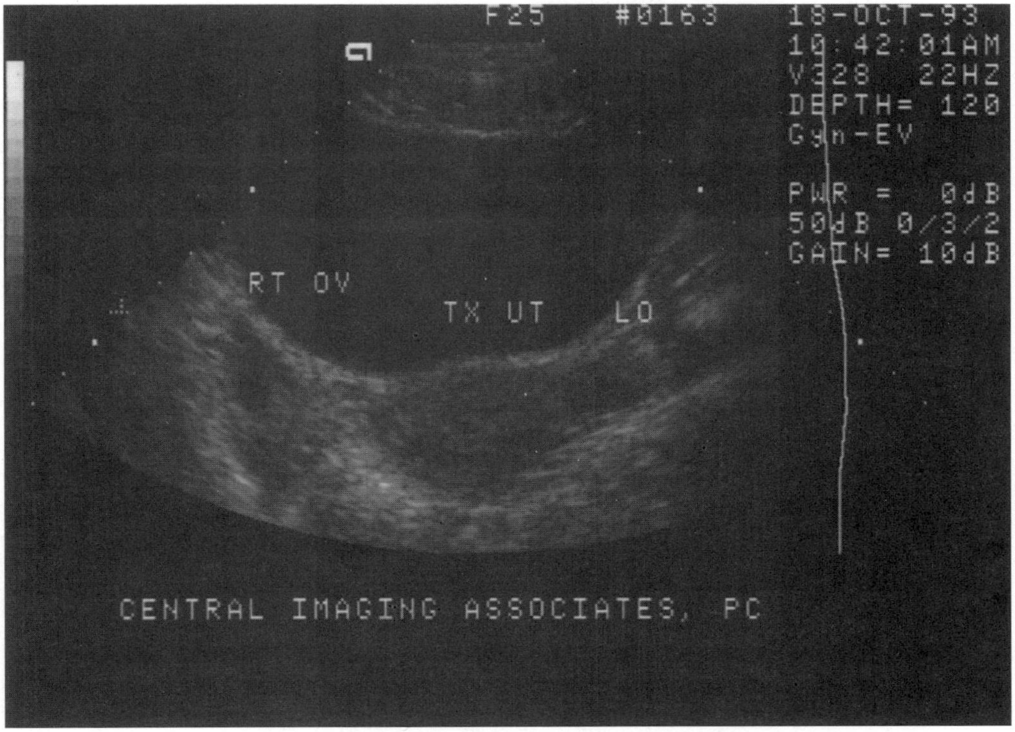

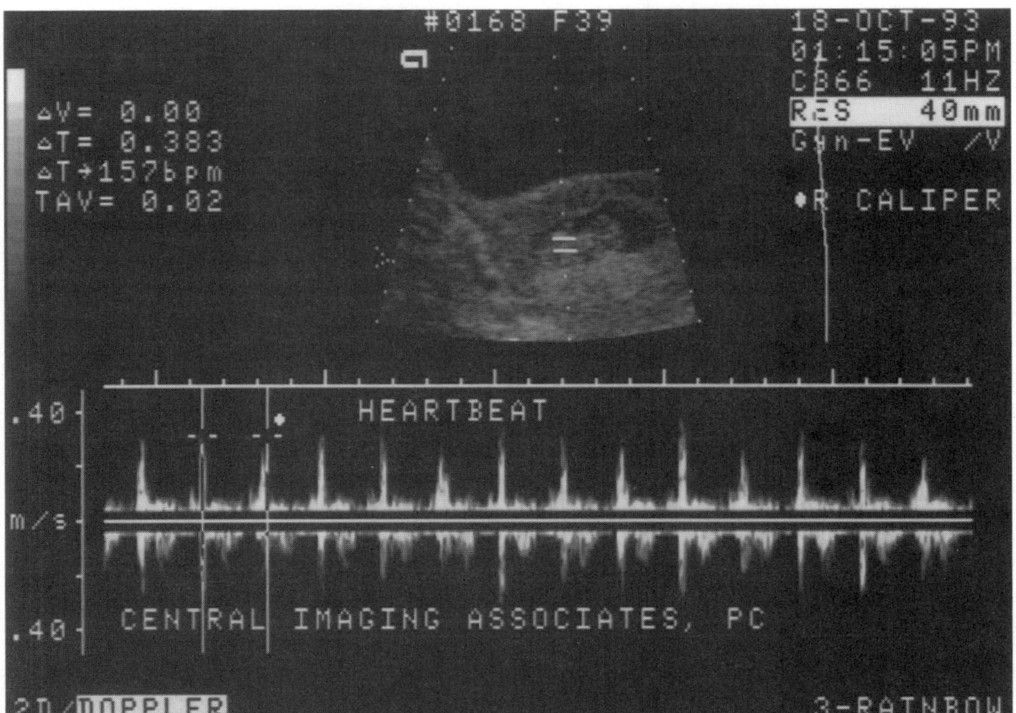

ULTRASOUND WITH DOPPLER

- detection of fetal abnormalities
- to confirm fetal life if in doubt
- to determine the presence of abnormalities which can be repaired in utero
- to determine the location and status of the placenta especially if praevia is suspected or placcartal demise
- to detect fetal masses

Gynecologically, ultrasound can be important. It can be used the following ways:

- to determine the presence of an ectopic pregnancy
- to look for the presence of a hydatidiform mole
- to examine the causes of abnormal vaginal bleeding
- to look for the presence of tumor/fibroids

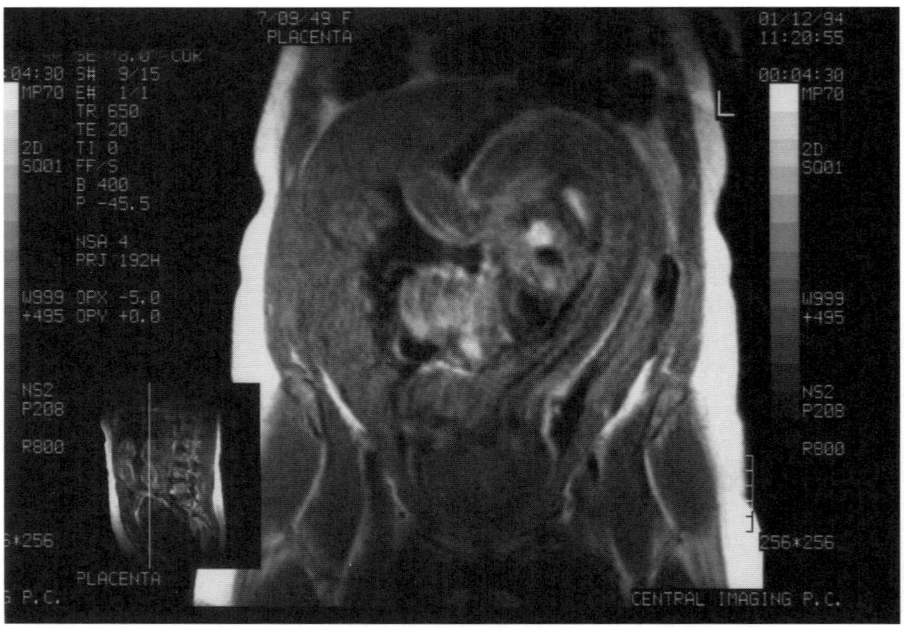

MAGNETIC RESONANCE IMAGING
TERM PREGNANCY (NOTE CERVICAL LORDOSIS)

GENETIC SCREENING

Amniocentesis

Amniocentesis is a procedure whereby the obstetrician aspirates amniotic fluid at approximately 14 weeks to determine the genetic status of the fetus. It is performed under ultrasound so that the practitioner can establish the position, the age and location of the amniotic fluid. The fluid is withdrawn and grossly examined as to the color and content. Dark red color usually presages some type of previous bleeding episode and the likelihood of previous fetal trauma is great. Bright red blood however may indicate maternal puncture and be non-important. The safety of this procedure has been in question for many years. Tabor et.al demonstrated in a large randomized trial study that the possibility of miscarriage after amniocentesis is approximately 0.5%. This is quite high when one considers the number of defects they uncover. In addition there is the possibility of a false positive or false negative result thus misinforming the prospective parents. The lay person most often considers amniocentesis for the older mother who is at greater risk for giving birth to a Down's syndrome child. When asked about amniocentesis in the office we often recommend that if the parents are likely to terminate the pregnancy based upon the data they receive than the test has merit. Should they not consider an alternative to the pregnancy, then the test will serve only to concern them should there be a positive result.

A recent study has shown that children born to mothers who have amniocentesis in utero have a higher incidence of "unexplained" bilateral otitis media through childhood. While medical doctors may not see the relevance, chiropractors can understand this more easily in relation to the pressures on the developing bony skeleton especially that of the cranial bones. While the amniotic fluid replenishes itself for a period of time the pressure gradient in utero is changing. This change may be enough to alter the position of the cranial bones sufficiently to cause an alteration in the attitude of the eustachian tubes in the baby thus impeding drainage.

Chronic villus sampling

CVS sampling can be done by inserting a catheter into the placenta by means of the abdomen, cervix or vagina. As with amniocentesis it is done under ultrasound and carries the same effects as does amniocentesis. The spontaneous abortion rate as a result of CVS sampling is approximately 0.8%.

These procedures are quite popular among obstetricians for many reasons, some of the more important considerations for their use being:

1) Parents who have had a previous child with a genetic abnormality
2) Age of the mother

NUTRITION

Nutrition has a significant effect on the outcome of a pregnancy. Much theoretical consideration is presently being given to the possibility of malnutrition as the major cause of toxemia in pregnancy. History contains many instances where whole populations have suffered either changes in numbers of births or in the health of the babies born. During World War II Holland had significant decrease in food supplies, and there was a 50% reduction in the number of menstruating females. This reduced the number of births in total as well as the number of normal births. The types of problems that resulted from this malnutrition included everything from stillbirths and premature births to malformations of the CNS.

As we saw in Chapter 2 there is a significant weight gain that occurs during pregnancy, as a function of the hormonal changes and the changes that occur in the organ systems. In order to support the weight gain a significant alteration in the caloric intake needs to occur. There have been significant disputes in recent years as to the correct level of weight gain during pregnancy. Until recently anything more than an increase of 25 lbs. was considered detrimental to the mother and the fetus. These restrictions are now somewhat relaxed and other factors such as nutritional status and stature are also taken into consideration when determining the appropriate weight gain for the mother.

The weight gain in the mother is the result of an increase in the size of the fetus, the maternal organs, and the interstitial fluid, as well as an increase in protein and fat storage. Figure 3 shows the non-pregnant woman compared to a 24 week pregnant woman of the same stature.

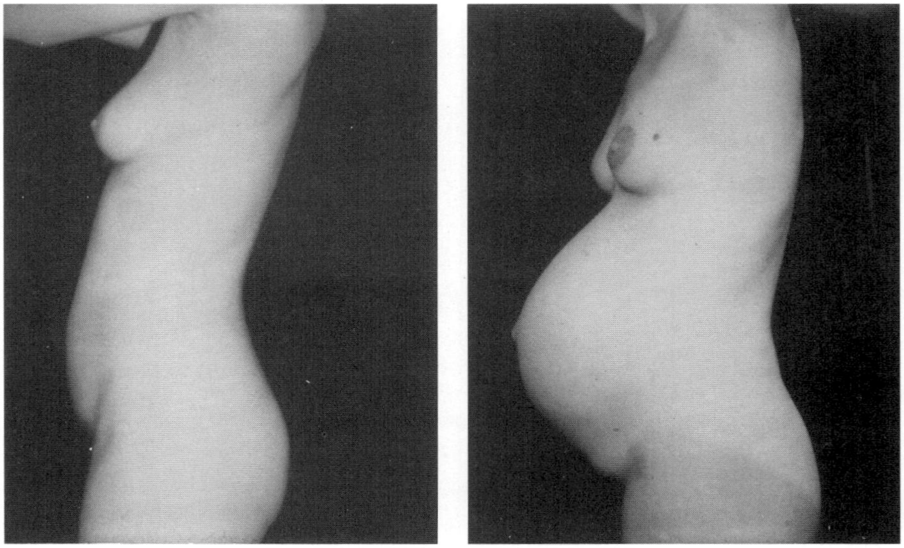

FIGURE 3

The overall weight gain begins in the first trimester and at that juncture is solely a response to an increase in eating patterns. The second trimester weight gain is accounted for by an increase in all the supporting structures in the mother and the third trimester gain comes directly from the growth of the fetus.

This weight gain has a significant effect on the lordosis of the spine, and thus will affect the overall subluxation picture in the pregnant woman. Weight gain in general will often induce subluxation and this is especially true in the pregnant woman when it is coupled with hormonal changes. High levels of weight gain are tolerated better by women who are in better physical condition than in those who are not. Strong abdominal musculature and good cardiovascular conditioning will predispose the pregnant woman to minimal effects of the lordotic changes in pregnancy.

One of the most commonly asked questions during pregnancy is, can a woman effectively remain a vegetarian and have a healthy child? Assuming that the vegetarian, whether lacto-ovo or vegan has a full complement in her diet, the answer is yes, the vegetarian can have a very healthy child. One of the most important factors with vegetarianism is the consideration of all the needs of the body. Some vegetarians commit what is known as an "error of omission," whereby certain foods are omitted from their diet for lack of desire when they are absolutely necessary for optimum health. The non-vegetarian has a large number of foods to choose from with respect to their nutritional needs. For example, they may choose beans, meat, or dairy as a source of protein knowing that the meat or dairy constitute what is known as a complete protein. The beans need to be combined with a food such as brown rice to give complete protein. The vegetarian, especially the vegan must therefore carefully choose her foods and pay special attention to the ones which supply nutrients such as calcium and Vitamin B12.

Exercise

In general it is important for the pregnant woman to continue her level of activity as she did prior to pregnancy. If the mother is a marathon runner it would be best for her to continue running at a reduced pace which the body will dictate due to its size. If the marathon runner suddenly stopped because she was pregnant it would be as problematic as if the non-runner decided to become one during her pregnancy. Moderate exercise is recommended for the pregnant woman. There are some pregnancy videos on the market which will give the pregnant woman gentle controlled exercise that will strengthen her and keep her fit during the pregnancy.

If you have never exercised, pregnancy is not the time to begin to do so. If you already exercise then you may keep up your present level of exercise until the physical limitations of the pregnancy prevent you from doing so.

Before attempting any exercise during the pregnancy it is MOST IMPORTANT that the doctor of chiropractic instruct the patient to consult with her midwife or obstetrician about the safety of a particular exercise with relation to their pregnancy. Some "high risk" pregnancies may not be able to support certain exercises.

The following are some of the most common exercises done during pregnancy:

Pelvic Rock

Have the woman on all fours with elbows and legs slightly bent. Lift the sacrum and lower back toward the sky in a "cat-like arch". Once up in the air, allow the low back to return to the flat back position. This should be repeated 10-15 times.

This exercise helps to relieve the excessive strain on the lumbosacral ligaments that is created by an increase in lordosis.

Kegel Squeeze

In order to tone the pelvic floor, kegel exercises have become extremely important to the pregnant woman. While the cervix has ample time to become dilated and stretched over the presenting part of the child, the pelvic floor musculature must quickly react to the change created while the mother attempts to push during labor. Doing kegel exercises during pregnancy will help tone the floor, and ultimately help keep the area from tearing during childbirth as well as help to prevent the formation of hemorrhoids. The exercise is done by squeezing and releasing the pelvic floor musculature. If the woman has a difficult time visualizing what to do, ask her to start and stop urination. It is those same muscles which make up the pelvic floor. By starting and stopping urination, the woman has isolated the muscles necessary to perform the kegel exercises.

Teratology of therapeutic drugs

Most all drugs other than large organic compounds cross the placental barrier and therefore can affect the growing fetus. It is postulated that drug induced birth defects account for approximately 2 – 3% of all defects, but perhaps this may be higher when one considers unknown environmental effects. Birth defects that present in a child at term are present in approximately 10-12% of all births.

From the 30th day after menstruation to day 75 is the period when the developing fetus can be susceptible to major teratogenic effects of drugs. During this time the woman may not know she is pregnant and continues taking the drugs. When she realizes that she is pregnant the effects of the drugs may already be expressed in the fetus. Of course the effects of therapeutic drugs may be expressed at any time during the pregnancy but some have been classically tied to early organogenesis.

Some classes of drugs that have produced significant deleterious effects on the growing fetus are:

1) Antiepileptic drugs
    - valproic acid
    - phenytoin
    - trimethadione
2) Antidepressants
    - lithium
    - tranquilizers
3) Antihistamines
4) Aspirin
5) Antibiotics
6) Cardiovascular Drugs
   Social Drugs
    - Alcohol
    - Caffeine
    - Aspartame
    - Smoking
    - Cocaine/Marijuana, etc.

Breast cancer and pregnancy

Approximately 50,000 women and 350 men develop breast cancer each year. Traditionally, only a small portion of breast cancers occurred before the age of 40, but now the number of young women developing breast cancer is on the rise. There are many causative factors which predispose a woman to developing breast cancer such as: family history, ethnicity, hormonal, diets, radiation/chemical exposure, alcohol/drug exposure, and other factors which have yet to be confirmed. With a family history of breast cancer the likelihood of developing a breast cancer prior to the age of 40 is increased. It is thought that there is a hormonal link in these cases with an increased level of estrogen present in the woman's system. This can be signified by the presence of an early menarche, a late menopause, late or no pregnancies.

Since the proper medical protocol calls for the routine removal of all lumps present, it is important that there is a breast examination before pregnancy to determine a norm for the woman. A proper breast examination includes a palpatory examination of the breast, a mammography, an ultrasonography and thermography. Each has a very valuable place in the diagnosis of breast cancer. Women do not often find themselves being examined in this fashion, and it is important that if one of the three diagnostic tests is performed that all three are performed.

Most breast tumors are classified as infiltrating ductal carcinomas and occur in the mammillary epithelium. In this epithelium there are estrogen and progesterone receptor proteins. Estrogen receptor positive tumors occur most often in the postmenopausal woman.

Breast cancer occurs in one out of every 3000 pregnancies. When they present during pregnancy they are more likely to be advanced than in the non-pregnant woman due to the late diagnosis. It is essential that a breast examination be done prior to or early in pregnancy so that should a tumor present itself, a baseline is established.

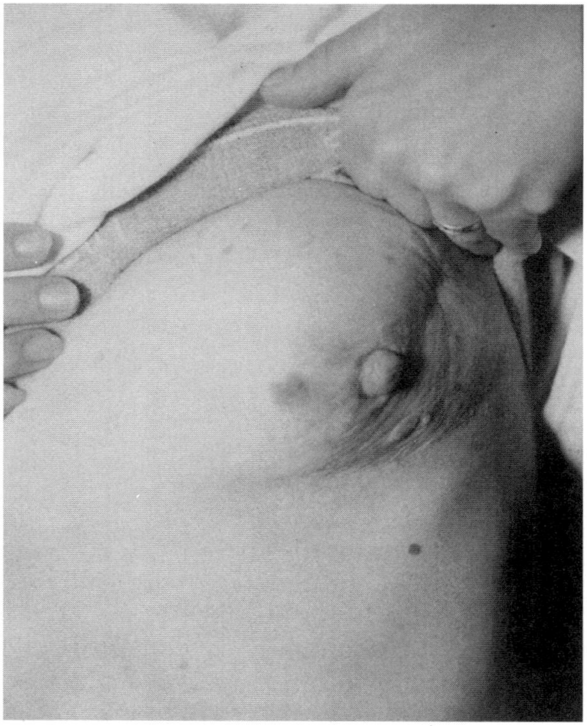

CANCER OF THE LEFT BREAST

FIGURE 5

Birth Plan

The most common source of unfulfilled childbirth outcomes is the fact that the preconceived ideas of the birth experience did not keep pace with the reality of what took place in the delivery room, birthing center or home. It is imperative that the pregnant woman have a very specific birth plan that is written prior to delivery which details the expectations and outcomes of the pregnancy. If her expectations are clearly delineated and agreed upon with the caregiver, then the likelihood of a poor outcome is minimized. Those things which should be clearly defined in the birth plan are:

Choice of caregiver

- obstetrician
- certified nurse-midwife
- lay mid-wife

Other Practitioners

- chiropractor
- pediatrician
- massage therapist
- acupuncturist

Birth Venue

- Hospital birthing room/ chair delivery room
- home
- birthing center

Pre-natal care

- frequency of visits
- level of invasiveness at each visit

Pre-natal testing

- ultrasound frequency/ abdominal vs. transvaginal
- amniocentesis
- CV sampling
- alfa-feto protein
- non-stress test
- other blood tests

Levels of activity during the pregnancy

- working outside the home
- working in the home
- other children
- exercise

What is your view on:

- anesthesia during birth
- what is your C-section rate
- how do you feel about VBAC
- how do you feel about childbirth classes
- how do you feel about nursing
- how do you feel about testing in women over 30

Labor

- how long to stay home before attending birth venue?
- how long can I labor before intervention?
- when would pitocin be used? level of monitoring during labor
- IV
- what positions can I assume?
- how mobile can I be?
- can I eat?
- under what circumstances would a C-section be performed?
- would you deliver a breech vaginal?

Medications during labor

- epidural
- anesthesia
- IV drugs

Birth

- can siblings be present?
- can my husband/labor support person be with me the whole time?
- how long can I push?
- what signals will you have to do a C-section?
- can I hold the baby directly after the birth before weighing etc.?

- will you be there the entire time?
- how often do you do an episiotomy?

Postpartum

- can the baby room-in?
- who can visit the baby?
- what will the baby eat immediately after birth?
- can I begin to nurse immediately?
- frequency of visits
- which pediatrician will see the child?
- when can we go home after the birth?
- given a C-section, how long in the hospital?
- should something be wrong with the child, what type of services does the hospital offer?

These are just some of the basic questions that should be part of any woman's birth plan. Again it is essential that she have her plan clearly outlined with respect to what she has in her mind for the entire pregnancy. If you couple a good birth plan with good pre-natal care and education, the birth outcome that is within the realm of human possibility will most likely be assured. ■

REFERENCES

Breast Cancer

Harris JR, Rechet A, Connally et.al: Conservative surgery and radiotherapy for early breast cancer. Cancer, 66:15427, 1990

Huguley CM Jr., Brown RL: The value of breast self-examination. Cancer, 47:989, 1990

Toxemia

Beck DW, Menezes AH: Intracerebral hemorrhage in the patient with eclampsia. J of Am Med Assoc, 246:1442, 1981

Chesley LC: The origin of the word 'eclampsia'. Obstet and Gynecol, 39:802, 1972

Gaitz JP, Bamford CR: Unusual computed tomographic scan in eclampsia. Archives of Neurology, 39:66, 1982

Gowers WR: A Manual of Diseases of the Nervous System. Blakiston Son & Co., Philadelphia, 1988.

Sheehan HL, Lynch JB: Pathology of Toxemia of Pregnancy. Williams and Wilkins, Baltimore, 1973.

Prenatal Testing

American College of Obstetricians and Gynecologists (ACOG): Technical Bulletin No.108. Antenatal diagnosis of genetic disorders. Washington, D.C. ACOG Meeting 1987

Cackle H, Wald NJ, Bankau G. et. al.: Biochemical screening for Downs syndrome. Lancet 2:851, 1986

Campbell S: The assessment of fetal development by diagnostic ultrasound. Clin Perinatal, 1:2,507, 1979

Fletcher JL: Update on pregnancy testing. Prin Care, 13:667, 1986

Glack L, Kulovich MV, Boner RC, et.al.: Diagnosis of respiratory distress syndrome by amniocentesis. Am J Obstet Gynecol, 109:440, 1971

Goldstein S: Vaginal endoscopy, Alan R Liss, New York, 1988

Rippey JH: Pregnancy tests: Evaluation and current status. CRC Crit Rev Clin Lab Sci, 19:353, 1984

Tabor A, Phillip J, Madsen M et.al.: Randomized controlled trials of genetic amniocentesis in 4606 low risk women. Lancet 1: 1287, 1986

Bleeding During Pregnancy

Cotton DB, Read JA, Paul RH et.al.: The conservative aggressive management of placenta praevia. Am J Obstet Gynecol, 137:687, 1980

Post D: Vasa praevia. Am J Obstet Gynecol, 104:151, 1979

Scott JR: Vaginal bleeding in the midtrimester of pregnancy. Am J Obstet Gynecol, 113:329, 1972

Effects of Therapeutic Drugs

Aase JM: Anticonvulsant drugs and congenital abnormalities. Amer J Disease of Children, 127:758,1974

Anderson RC: Cardiac defects in children of mothers receiving anticonvulsant therapy during pregnancy. J of Pediatrics, 89:318, 1976

Callaghan N, Garrett A, Goggin T: Withdrawal of anticonvulsant drugs in patients free of seizures for two years. N Engl J Med, 318:942, 1988

Diggory PLC, Tomkinson JS: Nausea and vomiting in pregnancy: A trial of meclizine dihydrochloride with and without pyridoxine. Lancet 2:370, 1962

Hartz SC, Heinonen OP, Shapiro S, et.al.: Antenatal exposure to meprobamate and chlordiazepoxide in relation to malformation, mental development, and childhood mortality. N Engl J Med, 292:726, 1975

Laegreid L, Olegard R, Wahlstrom J, et.al.: Abnormalities in children exposed to benzodiazepines in utero. Lancet 1:108,1987

Mujtaba Q, Burrow GN: Treatment of hyperthyroidism in pregnancy with propylthiouricil and methimazole. Obstet Gynecol, 46:282, 1975

Nakane Y, Okuma T, Takahashi R, et.al.: Multi institutional study on the teratogenicity and fetal toxicity of antiepileptic drugs: A report of a collaborative study group in Japan. Epilepsia, 21:663,1980

Rumeau-Rouquette C, Goujard J, Huel G: Possible teratogenic effect of phenothiazines in human beings. Teratology, 15:57, 1977

Safra MJ, Oakly GP:Association between cleft lip with or without cleft palate and prenatal exposure to diazepam. Lancet, 2:478, 1975

Ectopic Pregnancy

Barnes AB, Wennberg CN, Barnes BA: Ectopic pregnancy: incidence and review of determinant factors. Obstet Gynecol Surv, 38:345, 1983

Dorfman SF: Deaths from ectopic pregnancy, United States 1979 to 1980. Obstet Gynecol, 62:334, 1983

Loffer FD: Current concepts in the management of ectopic pregnancies. J Reprod Med, 31:73, 1986

Anatomy & Physiology

Austin CR: Fertilization. Englewood Cliffs, N.J., Prentice-Hall, 1965

Austin CR: Sperm maturation in the male and female genital tracts. In Metz CB, Monray A (eds): Biology of Fertilization, Volume 2, Academic Press, New York, 1985

Braude P, Bolton V, Moore S: Human gene expression first occurs between the four- and eight-cell stages of the preimplantation development. Nature, 332:459, 1988

Braunstein GD, Rasor JL, Engvall E, et.al.: Interrelationships of human chorionic gonadatropin, human placental lactogen and pregnancy-specific glycoprotein throughout normal human gestation. Am J Obstet Gynecol, 138:1205, 1980

Csapo AL, Pulkkinen MO: Indispensability of the human corpus luteum in the maintenance of early pregnancy luteectomy evidence. Obstet Gynecol Surv, 33:69, 1978

Eastman NJ, Hellman LM: Williams Obstetrics, 13th ed. Appleton-Century-Crofts, New York, 1966

Fallon JM: Orthopedic and neurological conditions of pregnancy, Multimedia Presentation, 1990

Fallon JM: The biomechanical and hormonal considerations of pregnancy as they relate to chiropractic care, Multimedia presentation 1989, 1993

Gill TJ III, Immunity and Pregnancy. CRC Crit Rev Immunol, 5:201, 1985

Grant JCB: An Atlas of the Human Body. 7th ed. Williams and Wilkins, Baltimore, 1978

Hearn JP: The embryo-maternal dialogue during early pregnancy in primates. J Reprod Fertil, 76:809,1986

Hunziker RD, Wegmann TG, Placental immunoregulation. CRC Crit Rev Immunol, 6:245, 1987

Knobil E, Neill J (eds): The Physiology of Reproduction, Raven Press, New York, 1988

Lenton EA, Neal LM, Sulaiman R: Plasma concentrations of human chorionic gonadatropin from the time of implantation until the second week of pregnancy. Fertil Steril, 37:773, 1982

Ludwig H, Metzer H, The Human Female Reproductive Tract. A Scanning Electron Microscope Atlas, Springer-Verlag, Heidelberg, 1976

McMullen M: Assessing cervical subluxations in infants under six months of age. Articles on Pediatrics Vol I. International Review of Chiropractic, 1994

Moore KL: The Developing Human, 4th ed. WB Saunders, Philadelphia, 1988

Pauerstein CJ, Hodgson BJ, Kramen MA: The anatomy and physiology of the oviduct. Obstet Gynecol Ann, 3:317, 1974

Scott JR., DiSaia PJ, Hammond CB., Spellacy WN. Danforth's Obstetrics and Gynecology, 6th ed. J.B. Lippincott Company, Philadelphia, 1990

Sholls HT, Orsini MW, Hitchins DJ: Estrogen synthesis and metabolism in the hamster blastocyst, uterus and liver near the time of implantation. J Steroid Biochemistry, 19:1153, 1983

Ulfelder H: Mechanism of pelvic support in women. Am J of Obstet Gynecol, 72:856, 1956

Wynn RM(ed) Cellular Biology of the Uterus, Appleton-Century-Crofts, New York, 1967

Exercise

Jimenez MH, Newton N: Activity and work during pregnancy and the postpartum period: A cross-cultural study of 202 societies. Am J Obstet Gynecol, 135:171, 1979

Lotgering FK, Gilbert RD, Longo LD: The interaction of exercise and pregnancy: A Review. Am J Obstet Gynecol, 149:560, 1989

Nutrition

Begner L, Susser MW: Low birth weight and prenatal nutrition: An interpretive review. Pediatrics, 46:946, 1970

Fahey PJ, Boltri JM, Mark JS: Key issues on nutrition. From conception through infancy. Postgrad Med, 81:301, 1987

Hemminti E, Stanfield B: Routine administration of iron and vitamins during pregnancy: Review of controlled clinical trials. Br J Obstet Gynecol, 85:404, 1978

Jarnfelt-Samisoe A: Nausea and vomiting in pregnancy. A review. Obstet Gynecol Surv, 42: 422, 1987

National Research Council: Alternative Dietary Practices and Nutritional Abuses during Pregnancy. Washington D.C. National Academy of Sciences, 1982

Piconce TA, Allen LH, Olsen PN, Fern MF: Pregnancy outcome in North American women. Ill effects of direct cigarette smoking, stress, and weight gain on placentas and on neonatal physical and behavioral characteristics. Am J Clin Nutr, 36:1214, 1982

Weight Gain

Abrams BF, Lans RK: Prepregnancy weight, weight gain and birth weight. Am J Obstet Gynecol, 154:503, 1986

Gormician A, Valentine L, Satter E: Relationship of maternal weight gain, prepregnancy weight and infant birth weight. J Am Diet Assoc, 77:662,1980

4 The Birth

The normal length of pregnancy is approximately 266 days from conception or 280 days from the beginning of the last menstrual cycle in women who have an average cycle of 28 days. This registers to approximately 40 weeks. These calculations are used only as approximations as only 5% of the total births occur on the expected day of confinement (EDC) or due date.

Labor, which is the event that ends in the birth of the fetus, is defined as the process whereby regular uterine contractions work to thin out the uterine wall and dilate the cervix resulting in the delivery of the child.

Labor is divided into four stages:

- Stage 1 - ranges from the onset of labor to the full dilation of the cervix
- Stage 2 - complete dilation of the cervix to the birth of the baby
- Stage 3 - from the birth of the baby to the delivery of the placenta
- Stage 4 - delivery of the placenta to the afterbirth recovery (4-6 hours)

The first stage of labor is characterized by two phases, one in which the effacement and early dilatation take place and one that encompasses the more rapid dilatation (Figure 1). The latter part of the first stage of labor occurs when the cervix reaches 3-4 cm. During this stage of labor, the progress is measured in amount of dilatation, the station of the fetal head and the amount of effacement (Figure 1).

Stage 2 of labor is characterized by the full dilatation of the cervix and the imminent birth of the child. The normal birth mechanism (Figure 2) is described by its cardinal movements of labor. They are shown in Table 1. (Note: Most commonly these cardinal movements are thought to range from 4-6 in number. For teaching purposes they are shown here in seven movements)1.

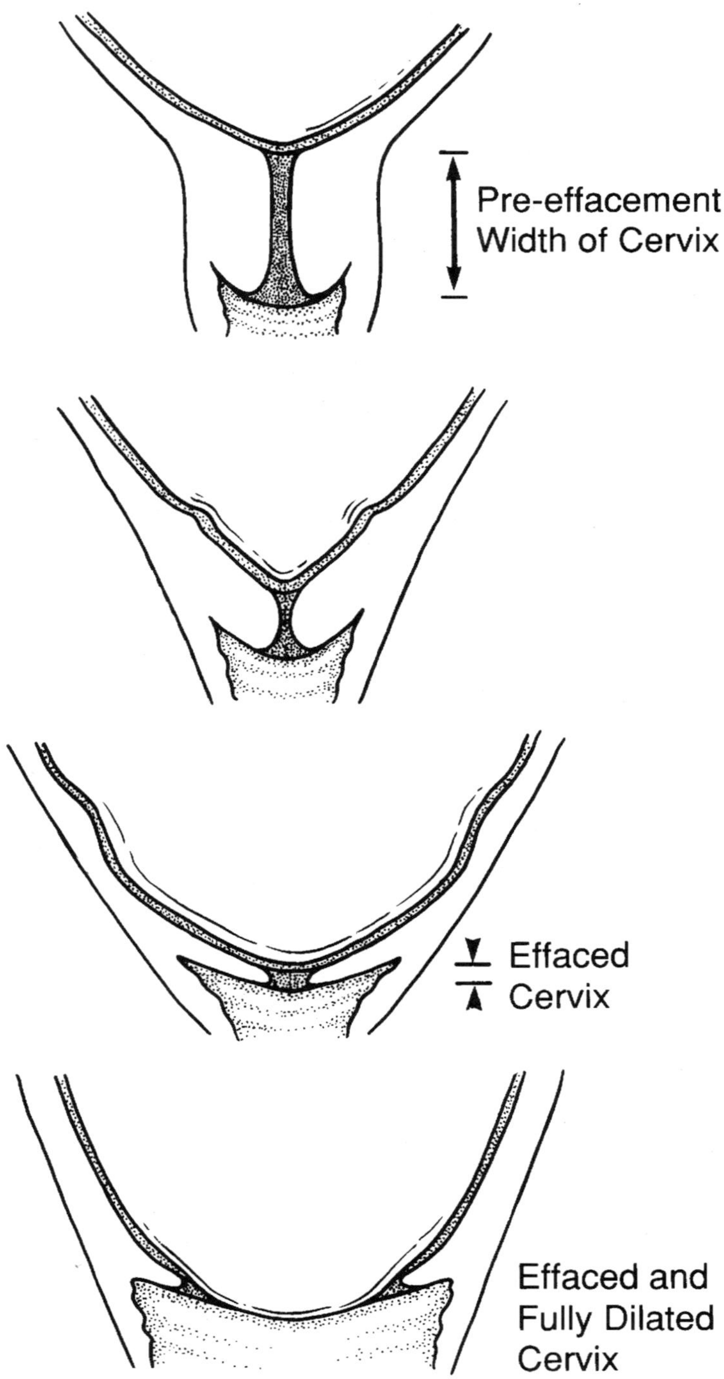
Pre-effacement
Width of Cervix
Effaced
Cervix
Effaced and
Fully Dilated
Cervix

FIGURE 1

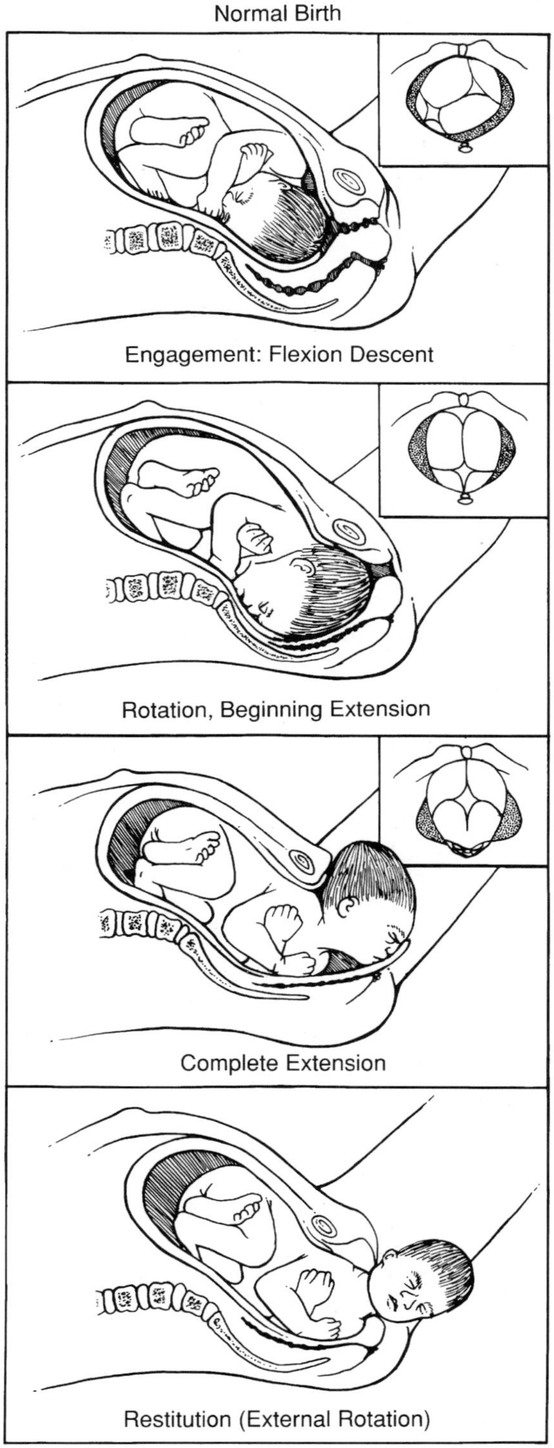
Normal Birth
Engagement: Flexion Descent
Rotation, Beginning Extension
Complete Extension
Restitution (External Rotation)

FIGURE 2

I) Engagment	V) Extension
II) Descent	VI) External Rotation
III) Flexion	VII) Expulsion
IV) Internal Rotation	

TABLE 1

As the second stage of labor begins, the force and need to bear down begins the descent of the fetus through the birth canal. Once the head is engaged, the fetus then begins its descent. As the uterine contractions bring the fetus downward, the fetus assumes a more flexed position. As the fetal head meets the pelvic floor, at station zero (level of the ishial spines) the fetus begins to rotate internally so that the occiput is anteriorly against the symphysis pubis. In an OP birth which will be discussed later in this chapter, the occiput will rotate to the posterior and will be against the sacrum. As the "normal" birth process is considered to be an OA presentation, over 75% of OP presentations will rotate to an OA. Extension occurs as the fetus continues its descent through the pelvis and crowning of the head will occur as the largest diameter of the fetal head reaches the vulvar ring, and the head is then born with rapid extension underneath the symphysis pubis. It should be noted here that this is the first moulding of the child's spine that occcurs. There is a cervical lordosis that is encouraged as the fetal cervical spine is moulded.

The third stage of labor which begins from the completion of delivery to the birth of the placenta is as important a process to the birth, as the other stages of labor. The placenta usually begins to separate approximately 5-10 minutes after the birth of the child. Tugging and pulling on the umbilical cord of the child to hasten delivery of the placenta is not recommended. If the placental delivery does not occur in a reasonable amount of time, gentle uterine massage may be applied to hasten the delivery. The placenta should be examined to make sure that it is complete and no part remains in the uterus.

The fourth stage of labor is characterized by close observation of the mother and the fetus. Vital signs should be monitored, and signs of excessive uterine bleeding closely watched.

Induction of labor

Sometimes a labor needs to either be speeded up or begun because of some type of danger to the mother or fetus and is induced by the hormone Oxytocin or some derivative the most common substance of which is Pitocin (Pitting). Some of the indications for induction of labor include:

- Premature rupture of the membranes where infection is a possibility
- Danger to the fetus/mother
- other

When a mother has had previous surgery on the uterus where the integrity of the uterine has been disrupted, there is a danger in inducing labor as the strong contractions the Pitocin may produce can result in uterine rupture.

Position of the fetus

The position of the fetus is determined relative to its position within the pelvis. Position is important as it may determine the type of delivery and the subsequent effects on the newborn. The normal presentations are determined relative to the following:

PRESENTATION

the part of the fetus at the lower pole

cephalic - face
vertex - occiput
breech - foot/buttocks

ATTITUDE

the position of the fetus relative to itself

flexion
deflexion
extension

DENOMINATOR

the part that presents

occiput in a vertex birth
foot/buttocks in a breech birth
mentum in a cephalic

LIE

the position of the long axis of the fetus relative to the mother

(L) longitudinal
(T) transverse
(O) oblique

Complications of Labor

The complications of birth can be divided into three categories:

1) Polarity (POWER)
2) Passenger (BABY)
3) Passage (PELVIS)

As one looks at the possible complications of labor it is easy to see that the chiropractor can have an enormous effect on the outcome. Helping the pregnant woman to maintain neuromuscular harmony (polarity) and ensure that the child has the proper nutrition, proper placement (passenger), as well as making sure that the pelvis is not subluxated (passage) can help minimize possible complications and optimize the birth experience.

Polarity (POWER)

The polarity of the uterus is essential for a normal labor. One can experience a normal polarity with weak contractions or an abnormal polarity where the contractions are disordered or parts of the uterus do not act together with the others. With normal polarity with weak contractions, the woman is likely to become exhausted due to the protracted labor time. This can increase fetal distress, and may lead to an ultimate C-section.

Abnormal polarity which ranges from disordered or incoordinate uterine contractions to cervical dystocia can also cause painful and unproductive uterine contractions and place the fetus in a position of distress leading to an ultimate C-section. The following are some types of abnormal polarity.

- Disordered uterine action
- Colicky uterus
- Constriction ring–Bandl's ring
- Rigid cervix
- Edematous cervix
- Annular detachment

Passenger (BABY)

Malposition, malpresentation, and multiple pregnancy, have all been discussed in other areas of the book. Each one of these may cause a problem with respect to the labor.

Passage (PELVIS)

Any osseous change which occurs in the pelvis can potentially cause a problem during labor. In addition, fibroid tumors or uterine malformation can also lead to an altered passageway for the baby. Some of the possible problems in this regard are:

- Tumors
- Cysts
- Fractures
- Physiological changes: DJD/TB/rickets/osteomalacia
- Flat pelvis/android (male) pelvis
- Subluxation

MALPOSITION

Malposition of the fetus can cause specific subluxations in the newborn. It is important to consider the changes that the fetus undergoes as a function of malposition. The malpositions are as follows:

Occiput posterior

Occurs in 13% of all head presentations where the presenting part is the vertex and the denominator is the occiput. Commonly referred to as being born "upside down" or "sunnyside up" (Figure 3).

Possible causes: pendulous abdomen
small pelvic size
flat sacrum
anterior wall placenta

Some of the more classic signs of an occiput posterior presentation is that there is usually what is termed "back labor," and the membranes sometimes rupture before the onset of labor. In women who have been adjusted throughout their pregnancy, back labor is usually non-existent and cannot be used by the obstetrician/midwife as a sign of posterior birth. The mechanism of back labor is that the head of the fetus is pressing on the sacrum, thereby causing pressure on the sacral plexus. When the SI joints open to permit the passage of the fetus in an OP birth, if there is sacral/SI subluxation, the presence of the head of the fetus causes significant back discomfort. In the OP birth where there is no subluxation, the possibility of back labor is minimized.

Under optimum circumstances the OP will change to an OA by turning 135° (Figure 4).

A persistent OP that does not turn to an OA or that turns late will produce what is known as a "cone head." A condition such as Caput Succedarum, which is scalp lymph drainage impedance can result from a persistent OP birth (Figure 3).

OP BIRTH

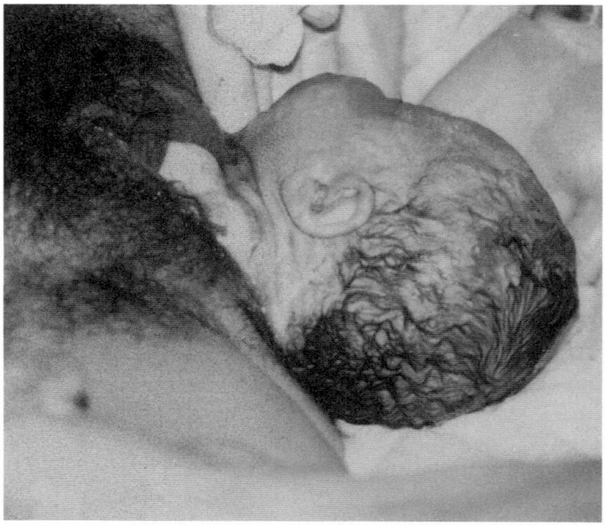

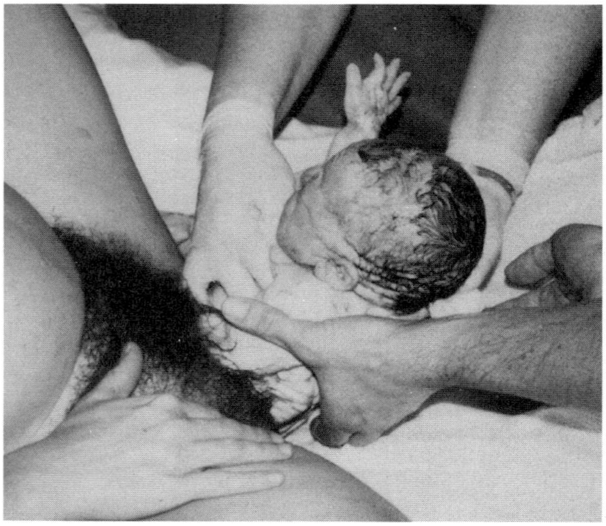

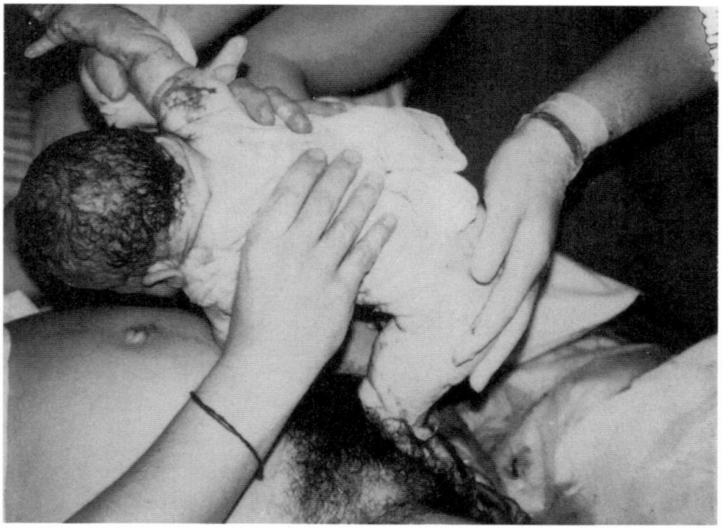

FIGURE 3

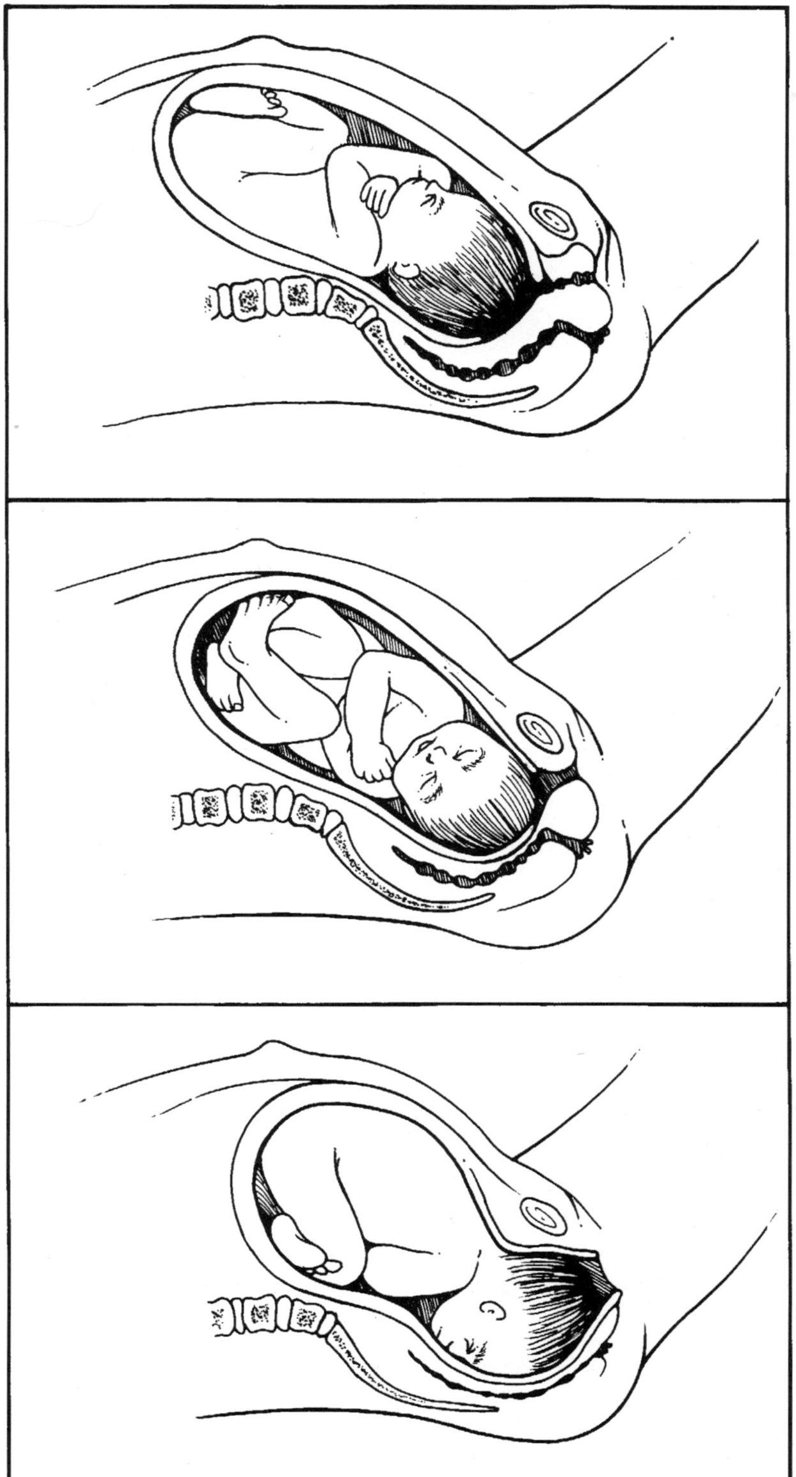

OP BIRTH–
135° RESOLUTION

FIGURE 4

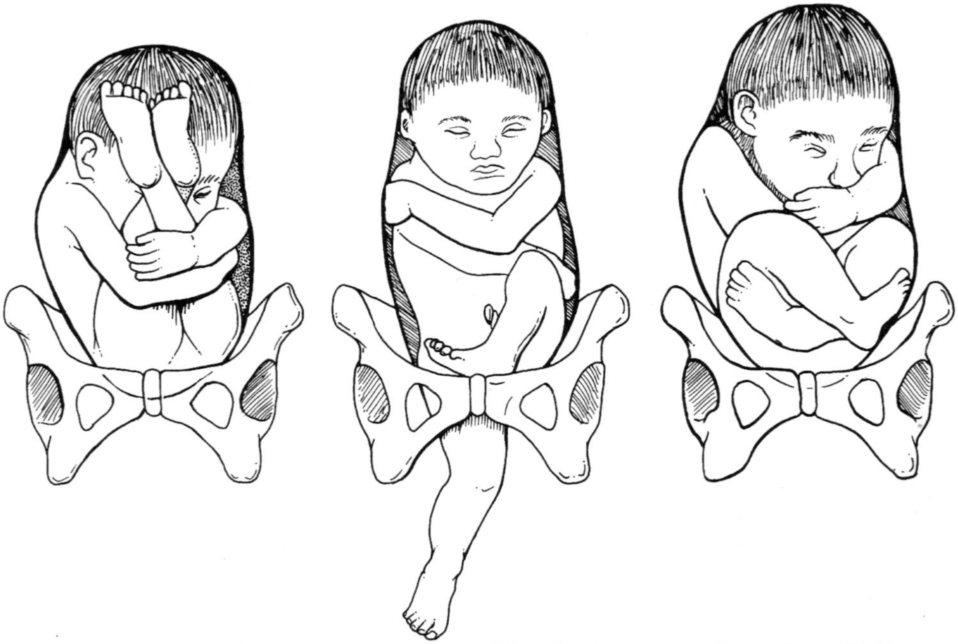

FIGURE 5 - BREECH POSITION

Breech

A breech birth is a birth where the head is not the presenting part but rather the feet, a foot, or the buttocks (Figure 5).

The breech birth occurs approximately one in 40 births, and is easily recognized prior to that time by the following:

- longitudinal lie with a firm upper pole
- hard head at the fundus with limbs to one side
- empty pelvis/without head

Due to the fact that the head is delivered last in the breech birth it is important to be somewhat sure prior to delivery that the head can pass through the pelvis. With other types of presentation, whether normal or abnormal, the first diameter that passes through the birth canal is usually the largest, whereas in the breech delivery the largest diameter is last.

Because of the risks associated with the breech birth, the R.N. midwife will likely choose to deliver the breech birth in a medical facility, whereas the lay midwife may choose to attempt the breech birth at home. The risks of a breech birth are as follows:

1) intracranial hemorrhage
   - rupture of the falx cerebri/tentorium
   - rapid moulding
2) dislocation of the neck
   - Erb's Palsy
   - damage to SCM (due to traction)
3) rupture of internal organs
4) genital edema
5) dislocation of the shoulder
6) fractured clavicle
7) uterine rupture
8) prolapsed cord
9) dislocation of hip joint due to traction
10) premature placental rupture/apnea

Face Presentation

Face presentation occurs in one out of approximately 300 births. The presenting part is the face with the denominator the chin or the mentum (Figure 6). This is usually due to a lax uterus, flat pelvis, multiple fetus, anencephaly or neck spasms of the fetus. Of interest to the chiropractor is the extreme extension that the child experiences who is born in this position. The occiput rests on the shoulders and there is flattening of the frontal bone. In addition, the SCM is stretched and the anterior musculature of the neck is affected. The presence of subluxation of the upper cervical vertebrae is readily apparent as a result of this birth. The possibility of this presentation should be considered when there is frank subluxation and abnormal moulding of the cranial bones.

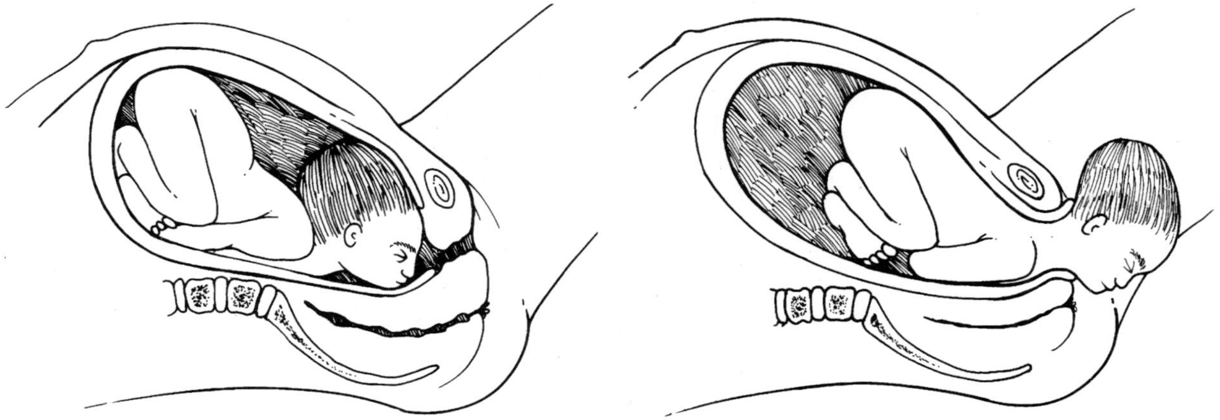

FACE PRESENTATION

FIGURE 6

Brow presentation

Brow presentations (Figure 7) are most often unstable due to the fact that A-P diameter of the head is too large to pass through the pelvic outlet. They usually revert to a occiput posterior or a face presentation. A persistent brow presentation can present with a significant compressive effect on the cervical spine. While the child is most often born by another presentation, the descent down the birth canal in a persistent brow presentation will most likely induce subluxation of the cervical or upper thoracic spine.

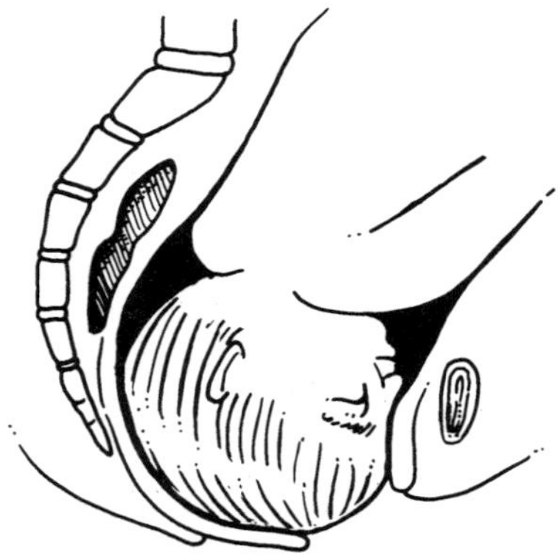

BROW PRESENTATION

FIGURE 7

Parietal presentation

Parietal presentation is found in the case of a flat pelvis and is an unusual occurence. The head is flexed with the parietal bone as the presenting part.

The parietal presentation (Figure 8) is a rare phenomenon and occurs only in the flat or platypelloid pelvis. The head usually engages in the pelvis with the saggital suture in the transverse position. This position is known as synclitic.

When the parietal bone is the presenting part it is considered asynclitic. In an anterior asynclitism the anterior part of the parietal bone pivots against the pubic bone with each successive contraction.

In a Posterior asynclitism the posterior part of the parietal bone pivots against the sacral promontory with each successive contraction and the head goes into extreme lateral flexion.

The most significant impact of this type of birth has to do with the lateral flexion of the fetal head and the pressure of the parietal bone against either the pubic bone or the sacrum. This mechanism may cause significant traction on the cervical or brachial plexus as well as compressive effects on the same. Immediate correction of this type

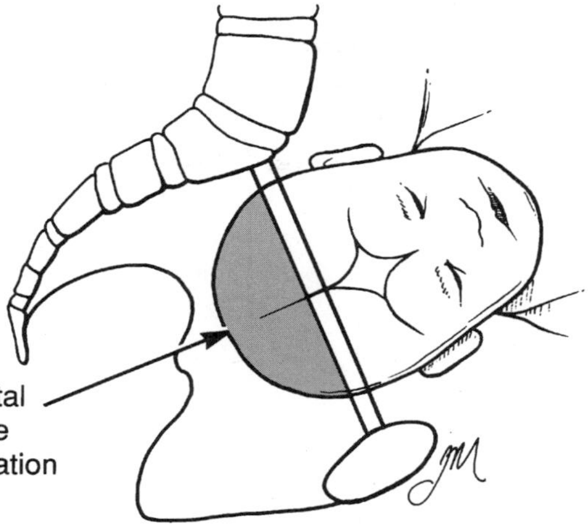

FIGURE 8

of subluxation in the newborn is most important so that permanent damage does not set occur.

Shoulder presentation

Occurring in approximately one out of 200-300 births, the shoulder presentation is rare and often converts to another more stable presentation. It is usually detected upon vaginal examination where an empty pelvis is revealed (Figure 9). The lie is transverse and the denominator is the shoulder (acromion). It occurs as a result of a variety of conditions including twin birth, hydramnios, placenta praevia, multiparity, sub-septae uterus, unusual fetal shape, and undue mobility of the pelvis.

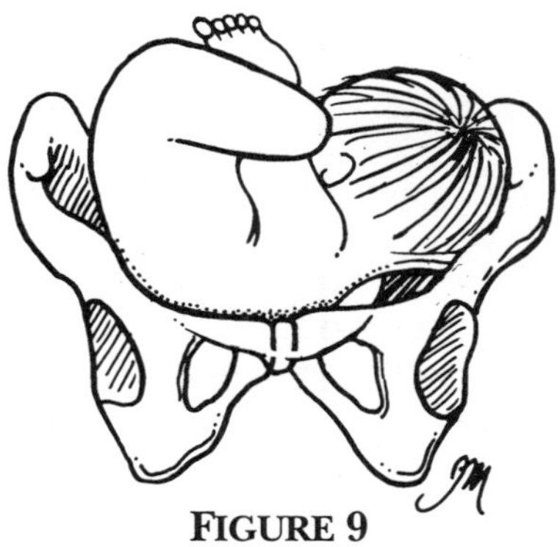

SHOULDER PRESENTATION

FIGURE 9

When this presentation occurs at a birth, one of the ways the obstetrician or midwife helps to allow for this delivery is to break the clavicle or the humerus to decrease the presenting diameter.

Compound presentation

Characterized by the prolapse of a limb alongside of a presenting part, with the nuchal arm (arm alongside of the head) being the most common of this type of presentation (Figure 10). Most often this happens due to malposition, malpresentation, small infants, or the lax abdomen and or uterus of a multiparous woman. This presentation is commonly known as "the baby fell out" syndrome of a woman who has had many births.

COMPOUND PRESENTATION

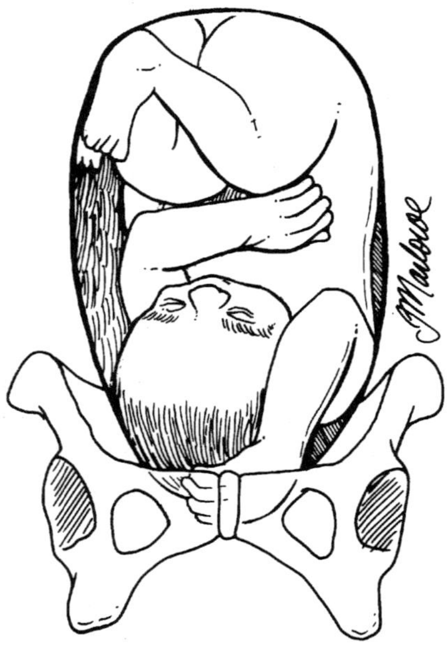

FIGURE 10

Forceps delivery

Although not used as much as in the past, delivery assisted with forceps is still a common phenomena. It is used when there is fetal distress, maternal distress, or a labor which does not progress favorably. Most obstetricians nowadays are keenly aware of the problems that the forceps can create, and try to use them only when absolutely necessary, and use them in the proper fashion. As we have seen earlier, a pudendal block is administered when the forceps are used.

When the head is high up in the pelvic cavity it is important that the practitioner not use the forceps. It is only appropriate to use forceps when the head is in the mid-cavity and a low-forceps technique can be employed. High forceps, which is a blind forceps delivery may result in injury to the fetus as the practitioner does not have any idea which part of the fetus they are grabbing. Should they make a mistake in the presention, high forceps may result in injury to the face of the child.

With the advent of more natural childbirth, the forceps have become a "taboo" instrument. As chiropractors we are aware of the extreme level of subluxation that they can create. Depression fractures of the skull, birth marks, iatrogenic torticollis and brachial plexus damage may result from a forceps delivery.

It is important to note that forceps are also used to help with the delivery of the head in a breech birth. In this case very often the practitioner will traction the head with the forceps in an attempt to remove the head quickly from the pelvic cavity.

C-SECTION

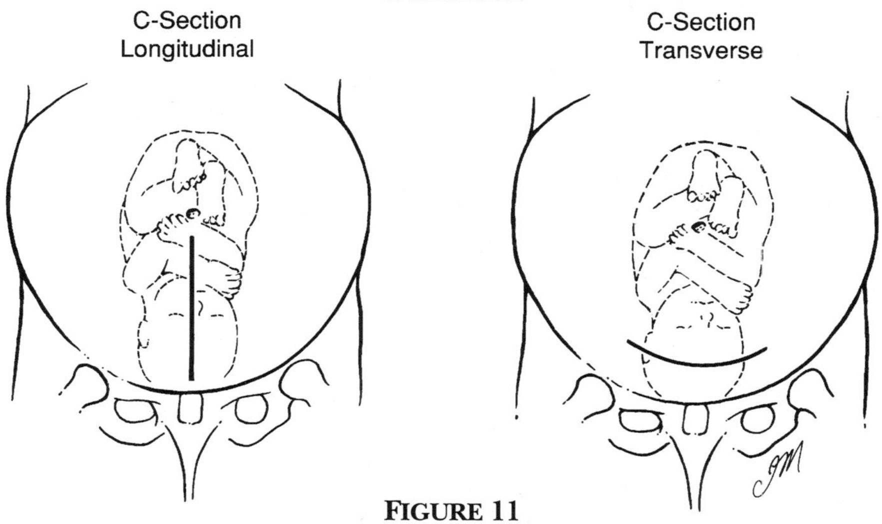

FIGURE 11

C-section

Often times when the labor does not progress properly or the mother or fetus is in extreme distress, it is important that the obstetrician perform a Cesarean section (Figure 11). Once performed routinely, it has become less common in the 1990's. Women have come to understand that unnecessary C-sections can produce problems for both mother and fetus and are keenly aware that a C-section should be performed only when another course is not possible.

The indications for a C-section are as follows:

1) placenta praevia
2) fetal distress
3) maternal distress
4) failure for labor to progress

A C-section is also performed at times for a breech birth and for predetermined pelvic distortion.

It is now routine for the obstetrician to transect the uterus in the transverse position rather than the longitudinal one due to the fact that the transverse cut heals more quickly, and reduces the possibility for subsequent uterine rupture (Figure 11). The old motto: "Once a C-section always a C-section" is no longer applicable, and the possibility of a VBAC (vaginal birth after cesarean) is now a reality.

Chiropractors are aware that the child born by the C-section does not have the benefit of proper head moulding. The moulding is important in the activation of the respiratory centers of the brain as well as in the expulsion of the contents of the lungs. It is therefore important to note that vaginal birth has important implications in the life of the neonate. Cesarean birth should never be considered unless there is absolutely no other alternative.

The healing time for a mother who undergoes a C-section is approximately 2-4 weeks whereas the mother who has a vaginal birth undergoes 5-10 days of healing. This of course does not preclude the postpartum period which occupies 6-9 months and often one year after childbirth.

VACUUM EXTRACTION

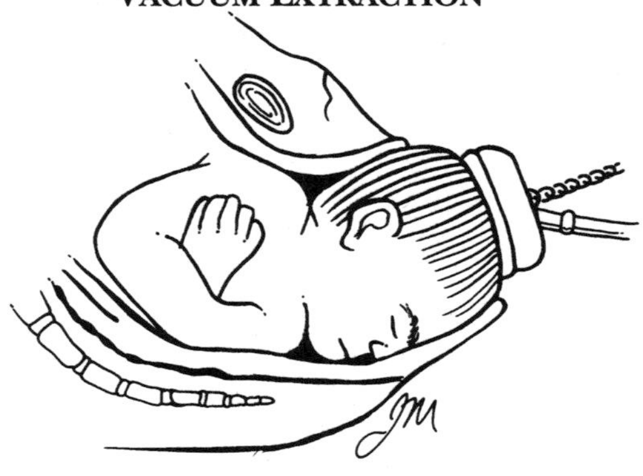

FIGURE 12

Vacuum extraction

Rarely used now, but sometimes used by the occasional practitioner, the vacuum extraction is used in much the same way as the forceps and for the same reasons. The suction cup is placed securely on the scalp of the child, and suction is applied to pull the head of the fetus out of the pelvic cavity (Figure 12). Sometimes when there is failure to fully dilate the cervix, the suction cap is inserted into the pelvic cavity and the subsequent suction will help aid in the dilation of the cervix.

As with the forceps delivery, this type of delivery is not without problems. The scalp, cranium and cervical spine of the child undergo significant stress as a result of this type of birth. Subluxation of the parietal bones almost always occurs in this type of birth and a cone head may also result.

Version

Version is defined as turning of the fetus in utero to secure a more favorable presentation (Figure 13). It is most often used to turn the breech baby to a vertex presentation. The most common move that is done is known as a Leopold's maneuver, and is performed usually under ultrasound at approximately 34 weeks. Historically this maneuver has been done in many ways ranging from acupuncture, acupressure points, to turning the entire woman on her back. Sometimes the child is rotated in utero at the time of birth. In this instance it is done to turn the child from an occiput posterior to a vertex presentation. There is a window of opportunity in which this can be accomplished and it stretches from 32 weeks to 36 weeks. Before or after this time it is unlikely that a version will be successful. Most obstetricians do not attempt this move as there are likely complications including umbilical cord stretching and placement about the neck. The midwife is more likely to attempt this maneuver especially if she is likely to attempt a home birth. ■

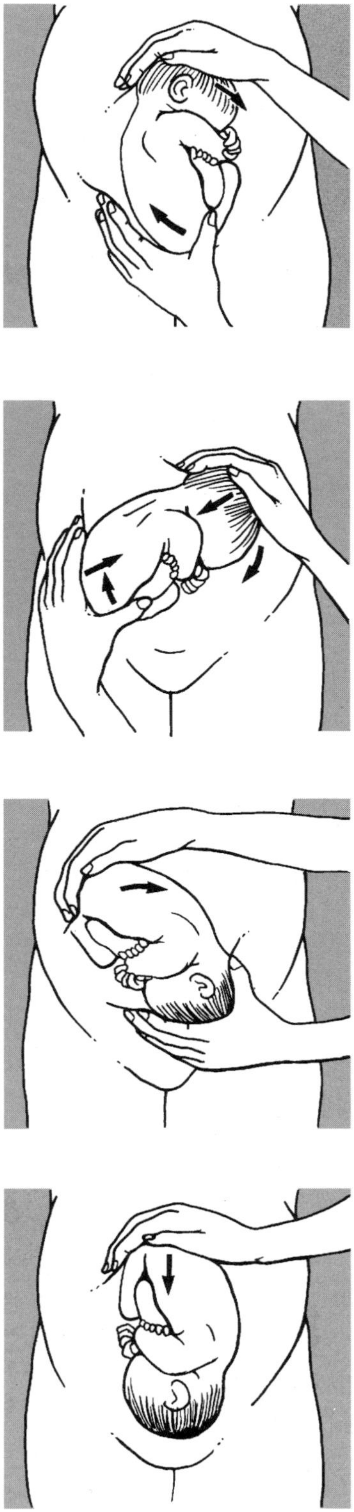

VERSION

FIGURE 13

REFERENCES

Post Partum Depression

Fondeur M, Vixsen C, Triebel WA et.al.: Postpartum mental illness: A controlled study. Archives of Neurology and Psychiatry, 77:503,1957

LLoyd JH: Puerpural insanity and the insanity of pregnancy and lactation. In a System of Obstetrics. Vol 2. Lea Brothers, Philadelphia, 1889

Robin AA: The psychological changes of normal parturition. Psychiatric Quarterly, 36:129, 1962

Zilborg G: Depressive reactions related to parenthood. American J of Psychiatry, 10:927, 1931

Operative Birth

Amirika H, Zarewych B, Evans TN: Caesarean section: A 15 year review of changing incidence, indications and risks. Am J Obstet Gynecol, 140:81, 1987

Bird GC: The use of the vacuum extractor. Clin Obstet Gynecol, 9:641, 1982

Broekhuizen FF, Washington JM, Johnson F, Hamilton PR: Vacuum extraction versus forceps delivery: Indications and complications, 1979 to 1984. Ob Gynecol, 69:338,1987

Caesarean Childbirth: Report of a Concensus Development Conference. US Dept. of Health and Human Services. Bethesda MD, NIH Publication No. 82-2067, Oct 1981

Dyson DC, Mellder PD, Armstrong MA: Management of prolonged pregnancy: Induction of labor versus antepartum fetal testing. Am J Obstet Gynecol, 156:928, 1987

Gibbs RS, Jones PM, Wilder CJT: Internal fetal monitoring and maternal infection following cesarean section. Obstet Gynecol, 52:193, 1978

Ryden G: Vacuum extraction or forceps? (Editorial) Br Med J 292:75, 1986

Taffel SM, Placek PJ, Liss T: Trends in the United States cesarean section rate and reasons for the 1980-85 rise. Am J Pub Health, 77:955, 1987

Breast Feeding

Anath J: Side effects in the neonate from psychotropic agents: excretion through breast feeding. Am J Psychiatry, 135:801, 1987

Behrem RE (ed.): Neonatal-Perinatal Medicine (2nd ed.) C.V. Mosby, St. Louis, 1977

Catz CS, Yaffee SJ: Environmental factors: Pharmacology in prevention of embryonic fetal and perinatal disease, Chapter 6. Washington: U.S. Govt Printing Office

Knowles JA: Excretion of drugs in milk: A review. J of Pediatrics, 66: 1068, 1965

Malpresentation

Amirikia H, Zarewych B, Evans TN: Cesarean section: A 15 year review of changing incidence, indications and risks. Am J Obstet Gynecol, 140:81, 1981

Bird GC: The use of the vacuum extractor. Clin Obstet Gynecol, 9:641, 1982

Collea JV, Rabin SC, Weghorst GR, et.al: The randomized management of term frank breech presentations: Vaginal delivery vs cesarean section. Am J Obstet Gynecol, 131:186, 1978

Cruikshank DP, White CA: Obstetric malpresentations: Twenty years experience. Am J Obst Gynecol, 116:1097, 1973

Dyson DC, Mellder PD, Armstrong MA: Management of prolonged pregnancy: Induction of labor versus antepartum fetal testing. Am J Obstet Gynecol, 156:928, 1987

Levine MG, Holroyde J, Woods JR, et. al. Birth trauma: Incidence and predisposing factors. Obstet Gynecol, 63:792, 1984

McMullen M: Assessing cervical subluxations in infants under six months of age. Articles on Pediatrics Vol I. International Review of Chiropractic, 1994

McMullen M: Handicapped children and chiropractic care (Part I, II). Articles on Pediatrics Vol 1. International Review of Chiropractic. 1994

Ryden G: Vacuum extraction or forceps? (Editorial) Br Med J 292:75, 1986

Taffel SM, Placek PJ, Liss T: Trends in the United States cesarean section rate and reasons for the 1980-85 rise. Am J Pub Health, 77:955, 1987

Systemic Changes During Pregnancy

Anderson LL: Regulation of relaxin secretion and it's role in pregnancy. Adv Exp Med Biol 219:421, 1987

Baird JD: Some aspects of the metabolic and hormonal adaptation to pregnancy. Acta Endocrinol (suppl) (Copenh) 277:11, 1986

Brody SA, Ueland K (eds): Endocrine Disorders in Pregnancy, Appleton & Lange, Norwalk, 1989

Chesley LC, Sibai BM: Blood pressure in the midtrimester and future pre-eclampsia. Am J Obstet Gynecol, 157:1258, 1987

Davison JM: Kidney function in pregnant women. Am J Kidney Dis 9:265, 1987

DeSwiet M:The Respiratory System. In Hytten FE, Chamberlain G(eds): Clinical Physiology in Obstetrics, 2nd ed. Blackwell, Oxford, 1991

Douvas SG, Meeks GR, Phillips JC, et.al.: Liver Disease in Pregnancy. Obstet Gynecol Surv 38:531, 1983

Easterling TR, Schumucker BC, Benedetti TJ: The haemodynamic effects of orthostatic stress during pregnancy. Obstet Gynecol, 72:550, 1988

Fallon JM: Orthopedic and neurological conditions of pregnancy, Multimedia Presentation, 1990

Fallon JM: The biomechanical and hormonal considerations of pregnancy as they relate to chiropractic care, Multimedia presentation 1989, 1993

Gant NF, Whalley PJ, Everett RB, et.al.: Control of vascular reactivity in pregnancy. Am. J. Kidney Disease 9:303, 1987

Grant JCB: An Atlas of the Human Body. 7th ed. Williams and Wilkins, Baltimore, 1978

Klein EA: Urologic problems in pregnancy: A review. Obstet Gyecol Surv 39:605, 1984

Lind T: Metabolic changes in pregnancy relevant to diabetes mellitus. Postgrad Med J 55:353,1979

Macfie AG, Magides AP, et. al.: Gastric emptying in pregnancy. Br J Anaesth 67:54,1991

Metcalfe J, McAnulty JH, Ueland K: Burwell and Metcalfe's Heart Disease in Pregnancy: Physiology and Management. Little, Brown, Boston, 1986

Milne JS, Howie AD, Pack AI: Dyspnoea during normal pregnancy. Br. J Obstet Gynaecol, 85:260,1978

Pritchard JA,Scott DE: Iron stores of normal adults and their replenishment with oral iron therapy. J Amer Med Assoc 190:897,1964

Smout CFV, Jacoby F, Lillie EW: Gynecological and Obstetrical Anatomy. Williams and Wilkins, Baltimore, 1969

Labor and Birth

Beazley JM: The active management of labor. Am J Obstet Gynecol, 122:161,1975

Beck NC, Hall D: Natural childbirth: A review and analysis. Obstet Gynecol, 52:371, 1978

Capso AI: Force of labor. In Iffy L, Kaminetzky HA (eds.): Principles and Practice of obstetrics and perinatology, John Wiley & Sons, New York, 1981

Carlson JM, Diehl JA, Sachtleben-Murray M, et.al.: Maternal positioning during parturition in normal labor. Clin Obstet Gynecol, 30:83, 1987

Danforth DN, Buckingham JC, Roddick JW: Connective tissue changes incident to cervical effacement. Am J Obstet Gynecol, 80:939, 1960

Freidman EA, Sachtleben MR, Bresky PA: Dysfunctional labor. XXI. Longterm effects of labor and delivery on offspring: A matched pair analysis. Am J Obstet Gynecol, 150:941, 1984

Ulmsten U, Ueland K (eds.): The forces of labor: Uterine contractions and the resistance of the cervix. Clin Obstet Gynecol, 26:1. 1983

Whittle MJ, Miller FC: The evaluation of uterine activity. Am J Obstet Gynecol, 136:38, 1980

Forceps

Freidman EA, Sachtleben MR, Bresky PA: Dysfunctional labor. XXI. Longterm effects of labor and delivery on offspring: A matched pair analysis. Am J Obstet Gynecol, 150:941, 1984

Levine MG, Holroyde J, Woods JR, et. al. Birth trauma: Incidence and predisposing factors. Obstet Gynecol, 63:792, 1984

McBride WG, Black BP, Brown CJ, et.al. Method of delivery and development outcome at five years of age. Med J Aust, 1:301, 1979

5 Orthopedic and Neurological Conditions of Pregnancy

Bell's Palsy

Bell's Palsy is a direct result of compression of CNV, the nerve within the temporal bone. It is most often seen in the 3rd trimester or during the postpartum period. All parts of the face are involved from the brow to the chin and it is usually unilateral. The patient most often describes paralysis of the face upon waking one morning without warning or any type of pain involved (Figure 1).

S/S
- sudden onset
- unable to close the eye, wrinkle the brow, purse the lips
- possible loss of function of anterior ⅔ of tongue for taste
- post auricular pain is present

Bell's Palsy in pregnancy was described by Bell in 1940 when he first documented the problem. Some of the most recent work describes it as having a possible viral etiology. Bell's Palsy is also seen frequently in diabetics suggesting a vascular component to the nerve involvement.

The most likely cause of Bell's Palsy is subluxation. Since MacGregor et. al. in 1987 pointed out that Bell's Palsy is seen three times more frequently in pregnant women than in non-pregnant women of child bearing years and older, it is most likely a function of changes that occur as a result of pregnancy (see chapter 2).

The author has treated 17 cases of Bell's Palsy in the office, 16 of which have been pregnancy related. Five of the cases presented during the last trimester and 11 presented during the post partum period. None of the women reported having had any type of chiropractic care during their pregnancy prior to being seen in the author's office. None of the over 300 pregnant women seen by the author has ever reported a Bell's Palsy. While this is hardly a representative sample, it clearly suggests that subluxation is most likely the prime etiology for Bell's Palsy during pregnancy.

BELL'S PALSY

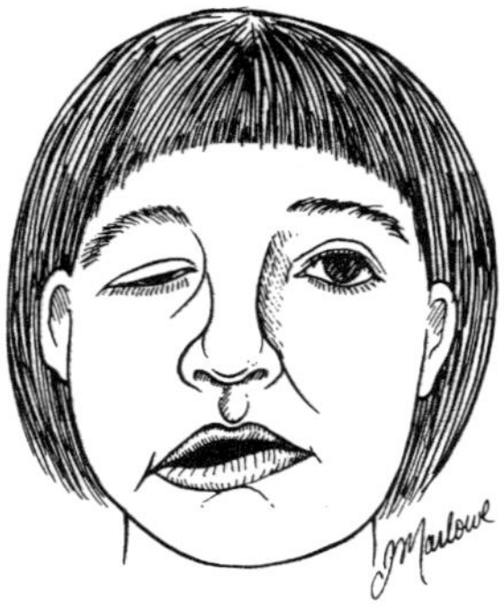

FIGURE 1

The mechanism of subluxation resulting in Bell's Palsy is postulated as follows:

- hormonal effects of progesterone and estrogen on the temporal bone and surrounding tissues
- presence of edema of pregnancy causing compression effects surrounding the temporal bone
- grimacing during delivery
- chin to chest pressure applied during delivery
- occipital/atlantial subluxation altering temporal position

Carpal Tunnel Syndrome

Defined as compression of the median nerve in the carpal tunnel of the wrist under the flexor retinaculum (Figure 2).

S/S
- painful tingling/numbness of the hand
- ache of the inner forearm with radiating pain

CARPAL TUNNEL

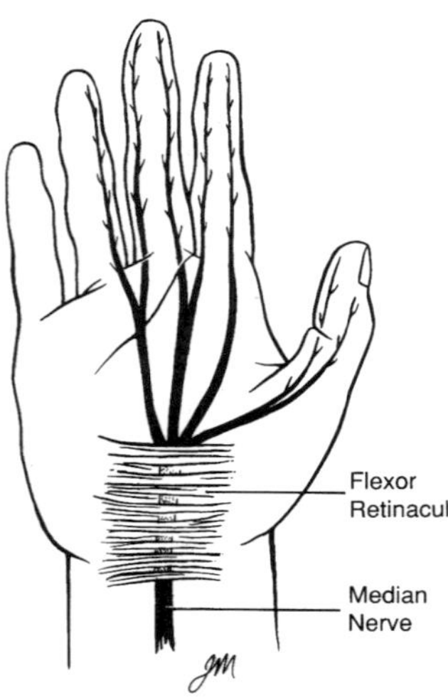

FIGURE 2

One-fifth of all pregnant women complain of pain in the hand (Noble et. al. 1971). Most have transient carpal tunnel syndrome, for as soon as the pregnancy is over the symptoms abate.

Test
- Tinel's sign - pain upon percussion of the flexor retinaculum
- weakness of flexor digiti brevi in the pinky to thumb apposition

Traditional medical treatment for carpal tunnel syndrome ranges from immobilization to steroid injection. These treatments bring only transient relief and they are most often not applicable to the pregnant woman. The danger of steroid injection and the impracticability of immobilization make the importance of chiropractic care evident.

Subluxation plays a major role in the occurrence of carpal tunnel syndrome especially in pregnancy. With the increased edema of the extremities and the hormonal changes, subluxation of the carpal bones is usual.

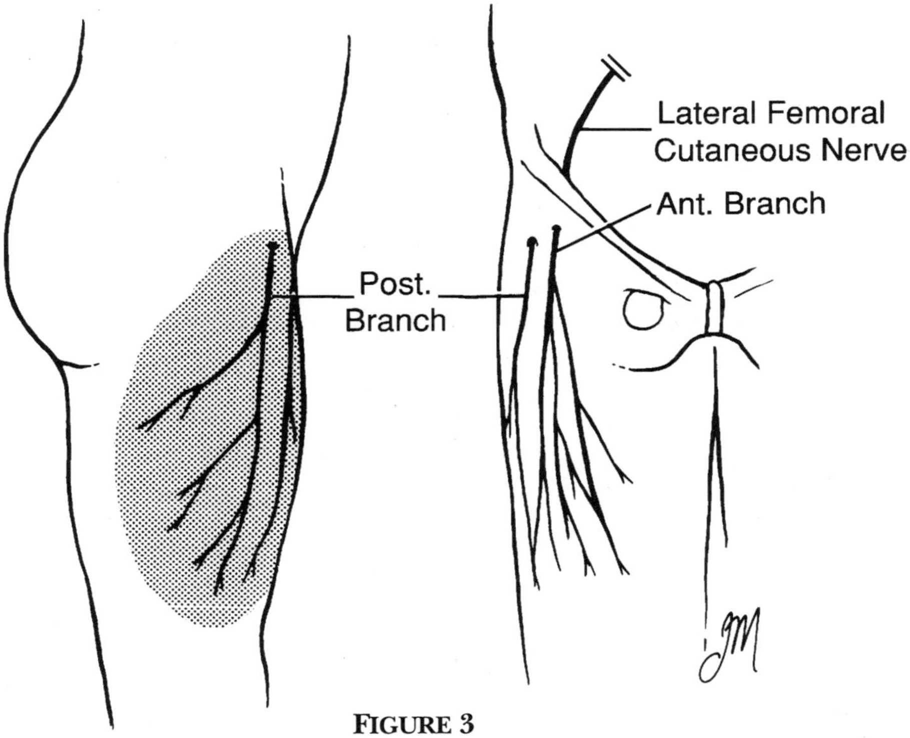

FIGURE 3

Meralgia Paresthetica

This occurs with the compression of the lateral femoral cutaneous nerve as it passes beneath the inguinal ligament. From the Greek *meros* meaning 'thigh' and *algos* meaning 'pain', the distribution of pain is classically in the upper thigh (Figure 3).

S/S
- numbness, tingling, pain in the middle 1/2 of the lateral thigh
- relieved by sitting
- exacerbated by walking
- begins the 13th week of pregnancy

Obesity and increased lumbar lordosis of pregnancy tend to stretch the nerve and this may result in it becoming compressed under the inguinal ligament.

NOTE: Inguinal hernias are common in pregnancy and rarely require surgery. Pain in the inguinal area should always be investigated relative to the presence of a hernia. Most often they will be bilateral and if they persist after delivery or symptoms of bowel strangulation occur during pregnancy, surgical referral may be necessary.

Separation of the symphysis pubis

One of the normal pre-delivery changes that take place in the pelvis is an opening of the symphysis pubis. When that opening becomes larger than 1 cm. it has traditionally been called a subluxation. The joint can open as much as 1 inch and is then referred to as a true luxation. The changes that happen in the SP joint will affect the SI joints as well and may cause subluxation there (Figure 4). Chiropractic adjustments to correct these subluxations work remarkably well in all circumstances especially during the pregnancy period. If these subluxations are not corrected during the pregnancy, they are far more difficult to correct in the postpartum period without the benefit of the hormonal changes.

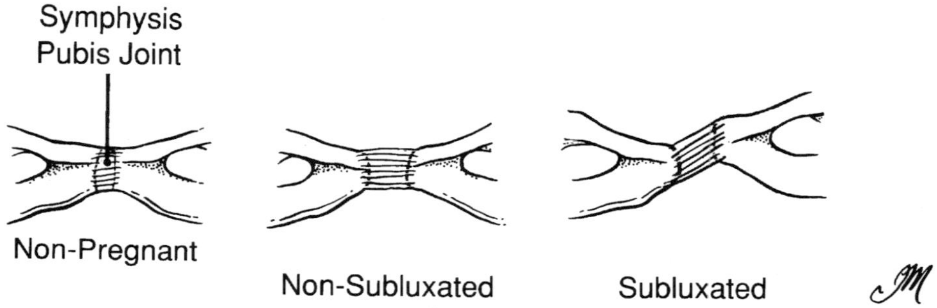

FIGURE 4

Coccydynia

Defined as pain at the site of the coccyx due directly to subluxation, this condition is seen after delivery but may be seen as early as the last trimester. Subluxation may be due to the increase in lordosis which changes the attitude of the coccyx relative to the rest of the body, or it may be due to a localized problem at the sacral-cocygeal joint. Due to its proximity to the ganglion of impar, subluxation of the coccyx may impart a myriad of symptoms unrelated to spinal disorders (Figure 5).

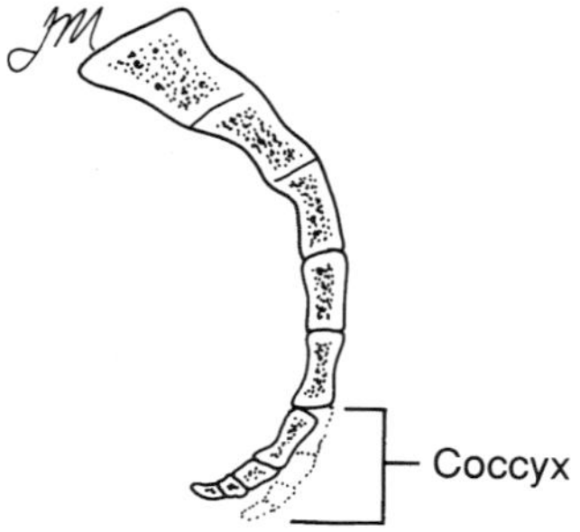

FIGURE 5

Very often the patient will present with a complaint that they would rather sit on a hard chair than sit on a cushion. This is classic with subluxation of the coccyx as the ishial tuberosities will contact the chair first on a hard surface and the coccyx will not come in contact with the chair.

Correction of coccygeal subluxations can be two-fold. One way is to contact the surface of the coccyx from the outside. If however the coccyx is tipped anteriorly, internal coccygeal pressure may be needed for the proper correction.

Sciatic neuralgia

Compression of the lumbar plexus results in irritability and pain into the buttocks and down the leg. This is by far the most common condition seen in pregnancy. Chiropractors know that this condition is classically caused by subluxation at one or more sights. The entire pelvis is capable of tremendous fluidity of movement during pregnancy due to the hormonal changes that permit it to open enough to allow for the passage of the baby.

There are two main levels of subluxation causing sciatica during pregnancy (Figure 6). Relaxation of the joint capsule, increased lumbar lordosis, and opening of the pelvic outlet with concomminant SI joint changes can produce sciatica neuralgia.

RULE OF THUMB: Women who have a history of back problems, especially sciatica prior to pregnancy will benefit greatly from the hormonal effects of "relaxation," and usually will experience less back pain during pregnancy. Those women who enjoy a healthy back and generally do not experience problems in the non-pregnant state will suffer from what they perceive to be a "lack of support" and begin to experience back pain during pregnancy.

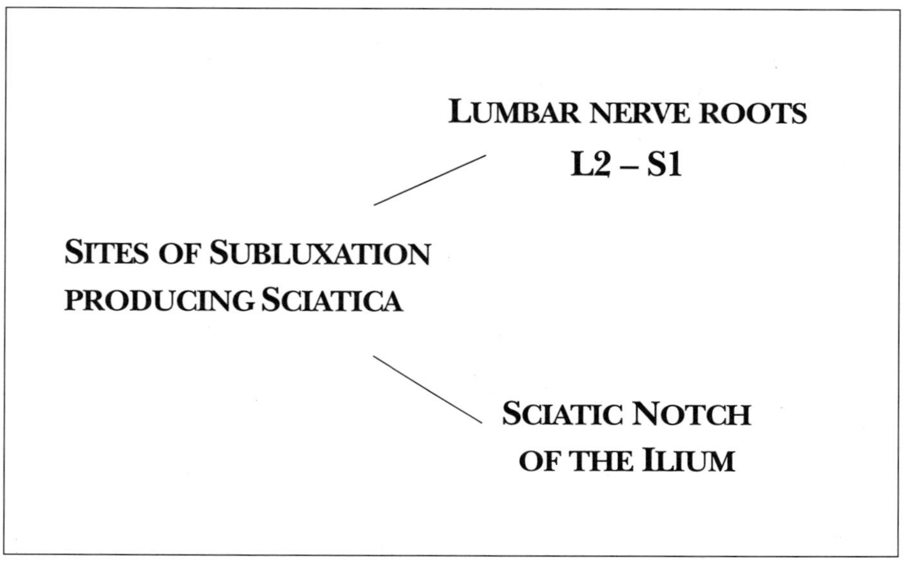

FIGURE 6

While the author has found this to be repeatedly true, it is also true that chiropractic treatment during pregnancy affords the patient the opportunity to correct conditions found in the non-pregnant state. When the hormonal effects are gone post partum, the correction made during the pregnancy is lasting.

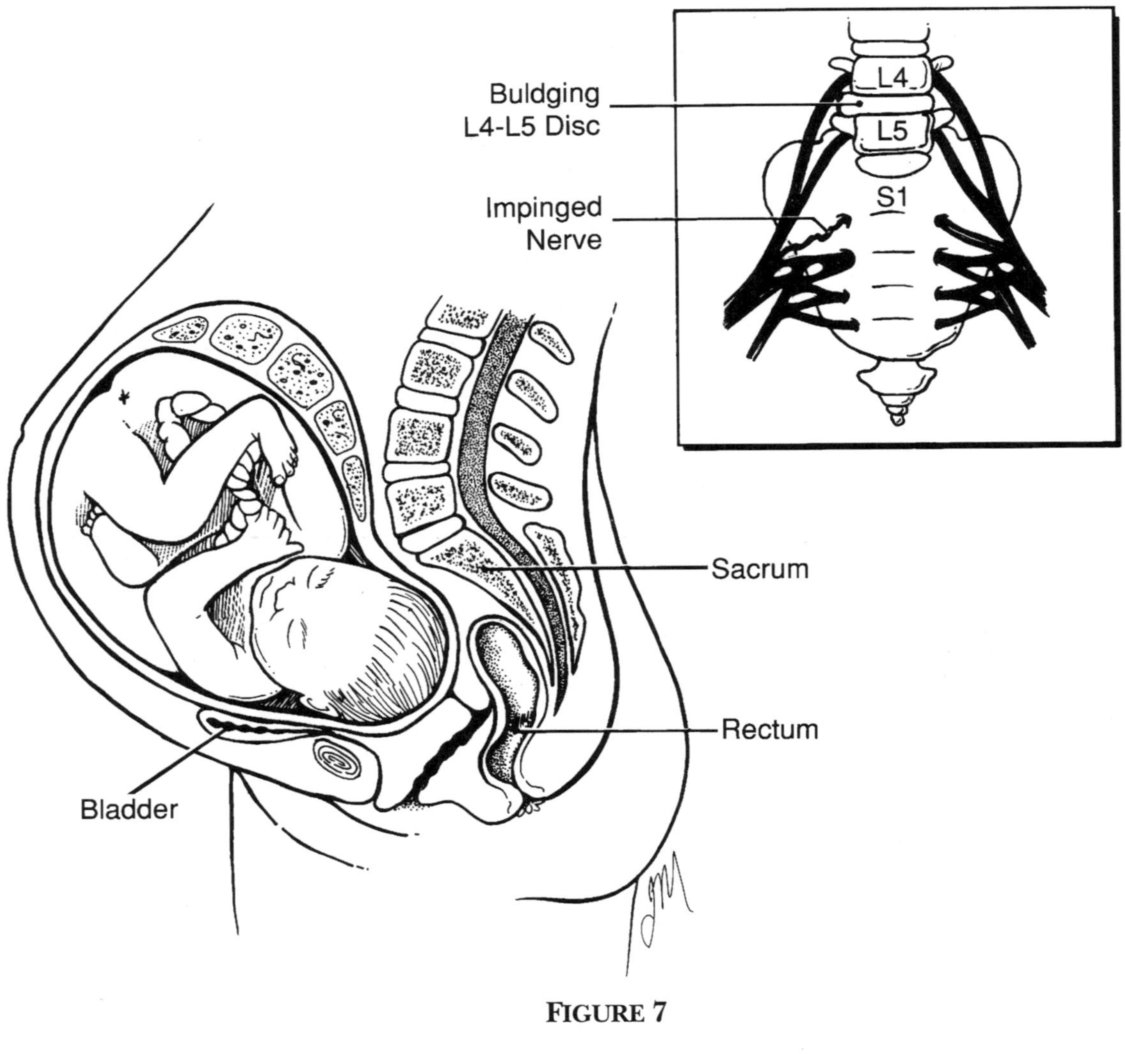

FIGURE 7

Obstetric palsies/traumatic neuritis

Motor or sensory deficits of L5, S1, S2 nerve roots resulting from trauma during labor or delivery, cephalopelvic distortion, dystocia, and primiparity are all causes of peripheral neuropathies (Figure 7).

OP can result from any of the following:

- disc protrusion at the IVF
- traction of the lumbo-sacral trunk (forceps)
- compression of the L-S trunk by the fetal head
- compression of the popliteal nerve due to positioning during delivery

The palsy can manifest in many ways with the following being the most common:

1) Foot Drop — Foot drop in the mother as a result of using forceps during birth was described as early as 1838 by Basden. In 1957 Brown and McDougall described a case involving a small primigravida with a large fetus requiring mid level forceps due to prolonged labor resulting in a foot drop in the mother.

   S/S
   - limp
   - weakness of ankle dorsiflexion
   - numbness and paresthesia of lateral aspect of the leg
   - a decrease in cutaneous sensation

These signs and symptoms clearly indicate that there is a sensory and a motor component to the injury.

2) Femoral Neuropathy — The femoral (anterior crural) nerve is compressed or injured during vaginal childbirth or C-section. L2, L3, L4 go deep into the pelvis and exit at the quadriceps. Attributed to strong flexion of the thigh onto the abdomen and outward rotation of the hip joint.

   S/S
   - unable to walk up stairs
   - can walk easily on a flat surface
   - decreased patellar reflex

3) Obturator Neuropathy — May be caused by a difficult labor where the L3, L4 nerve roots are compressed at the level of the pelvic brim.

   S/S
   - weakness of hip adductors and rotators
   - sharp pain in the groin
   - decreased perception of pain and light touch over the upper thigh

NOTE: Local anesthesia given during labor, called an epidural or "Saddle Block", may cause any one of these palsies by improper placement of the needle or torque applied to the meninges during the procedure. This possibility should be ruled out immediately as a cause of obstetrical palsy.

Correction of the palsies is dependent upon the nature of their cause. Subluxation may be at the root of many of these palsies. It is most important to take an excellent case history of the labor and delivery including what positions the mother assumed during contractions as well as during the actual delivery. Subluxation as well as deep compression or stretch on a nerve can result from a difficult or problematic birth. Given the proper questioning, a mother will be likely to give an insight as to the complete etiology of the injury.

Intercostal neuralgia

This is probably the first neurological condition to appear in pregnancy and is not always easy to correct as the hormonal changes coupled with the changes associated with the rib cage will contribute to the prolongation of this condition. Subluxation at the vertebral level as well as at the level of the rib heads can produce this pain. As the level of the rib cage changes and begins to flatten out, the intercostal nerves begin to experience compressive forces as well as stretching forces which produce change (Figure 8). Changes in the rate and depth of breathing as well as recruitment of the accessory muscles of respiration also affect the intercostal nerves.

Correction of the subluxation is left to each practitioner with respect to the type of technique used. Diversified, Gonstead, and simple double thenar moves are most often sufficient to remove subluxation at this level in the pregnant woman.

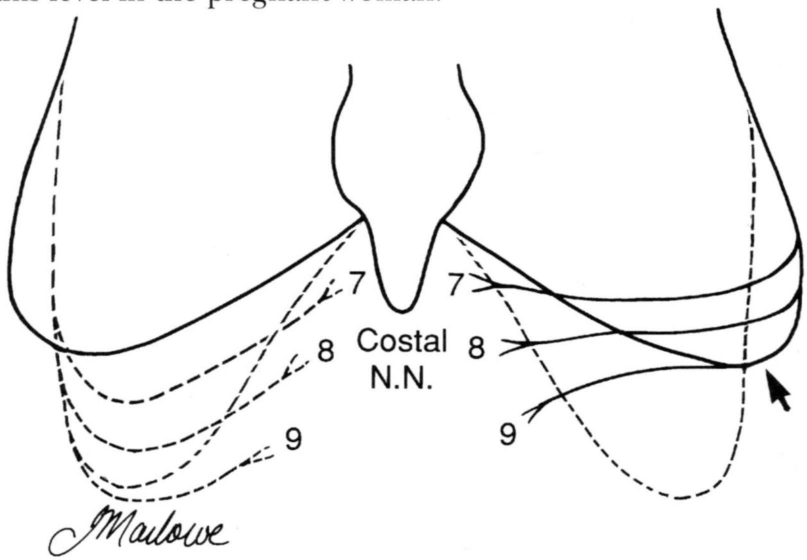

FIGURE 8

Brachial neuralgia

Compression of the nerves of the brachial plexus comprise this syndrome. Like many of the other neurological conditions of pregnancy, the hormones play a prominent role in the induction of neuralgia at this level.

S/S • tingling and numbness of the arm radiating down to the hand.

It is the radiation of pain that characterizes this syndrome. The impingement may be at any level along the course of the plexus which includes its nerve roots as well as its branches.

Correction of subluxation is usually performed at the levels of the nerve roots which occur in the neck. This correction will minimize the compressive effects of subluxation and correct the problem.

Headache

Of all the neurological symptoms that pregnant women complain of, this is one of the most common. Headache will be treated here as though it were a condition rather than a symptom. Most all headaches of pregnancy are muscle/tension-type headaches. Migraine headaches are nearly unheard of during pregnancy as most of those headaches have a vascular component which is minimized by the hormones of pregnancy. Somnncer (1972) reported that 77% of all migraines disappeared during pregnancy.

Most chiropractors know that nearly all muscular/tension headaches are subluxation induced. Applying all the principles of physiological change that occur during pregnancy, it is easy to understand how subluxation can induce headache.

Traditional allopathic treatment for headaches are not applicable to pregnancy for any medication can have an effect on the fetus. Therefore, chiropractic plays an important role in the treatment of headaches as well as all neurological conditions during pregnancy.

Lyme disease

No discussion of neurological conditions of pregnancy can be complete without giving some consideration to the possibility of the presence of Lyme Disease. Believed to be caused by a spirochete *Borrelia burgodorferi*, it is a disease which often presents with diffuse neurological symptoms.

Named for its discovery in Lyme, Connecticut, it is a disease which has its predominance in urbanized rural areas. The vector is a deer tick which lives on mammalian fur and is carried by mice from areas inhabited by deer to areas which are inhabited by humans. With the constant new construction that is going on, which creates new urban areas, the spirochete is now being introduced into areas that were once separated from them. With no place to go, the deer and other mammals are forced to co-habit with man.

B burgodorferi does cross the placental barrier. Markowitz et. al have shown that mothers treated for Lyme Disease have normal healthy full term babies. The author has treated over 300 pregnant women and the only miscarriage as a direct result of Lyme Disease occured in the 3rd trimester and was thought to be induced from vigorous antibiotic treatment. Once the symptoms have manifested even without signs of erthyema migrans, the disease continues to progress. The Western blot method of testing is the most widely accepted, but many physicians are turning to the Eliza method as it demonstrates more differentiation in the immunoglobulin levels.

When diffuse neurological symptoms present themselves during pregnancy and chiropractic care does not appear to have any effect, it is important that pathology be ruled out with Lyme Disease being an important differential diagnosis.

Pelvic neuromuscular stretch

Akin to Braxton-Hicks contractions which occur in the uterus prior to labor, the ligamentous and neuromuscular structures of the pelvis undergo a series of changes stimulating cramps which all pregnant women appear to experience. As the pelvic outlet changes shape and the SP and Sl joints widen, the ligaments and tendons undergo a series of changes which are classified by the author as Neuromuscular stretch. This phenomena should not be confused with the changes that lead to the various syndromes and conditions previously discussed. This is a normal phenomena that each woman experiences prior to childbirth, and is most marked in the 2nd trimester when the size of the mother does not equal in her mind the type of transient discomfort that she feels.

This level of symptomotology is most often treated as inconsequential by the obstetrician, and it is therefore the duty of the chiropractor to be aware of its existence and to allay any fears the woman may have about these feelings.

S/S
- cramping of the groin and buttocks
- transient leg discomfort akin to a "restless leg"
- muscle "pulling" inside the pelvis
- discomfort in the buttocks and perineum ■

REFERENCES

Neuromuscular Skeletal System

Adour KK: The bell tolls for decompression? New England Journal of Medicine, 292:748, 1975

Aminoff MJ: Neurological disorders and pregnancy. Am J Obstet Gynecol, 132:325,1978

Bell C: The Nervous System of the Human Body. Longman Rees, Orme, Brown, and Green, London, 1830

Berg G, Hammer M, Moller-Nielson J, et.al.: Low back pain during pregnancy. Obstetrics and Gynecology, 72:71

Berkwitz NJ and Lufkin NH: Toxic neuronitis of pregnancy: A clinicopathological report. Surgery, Gynecology and Obstetrics 54:743, 1932

Benson RC, Inman VT: Brachialgia statica dysesthetica in pregnancy. Western Journal of Surgery, 64:115, 1956

Brown JT and McDougall A: Traumatic maternal birth palsy, Journal of Obstetrics and Gynecology of the British Empire, 64:431

Cole JT: Maternal obstetric paralysis, American Journal of Obstetrics and Gynecology, 52:386

Ecker AD and Woltman HW: Meralgia parestetica: A report of one hundred and fifty cases, J Amer Med Assoc, 110:1650, 1938

Eckman-Ordeberg G, Salgeback S, Ordeberg G: Carpal Tunnel Syndrome in pregnancy. A prospective study. Acta Obstet Gynecol Scand, 66:233, 1987

Fallon JM: Orthopedic and neurological conditions of pregnancy and chiropractic management of care, Articles on Pediatrics, International Review of Chiropractic Vol II, 1994

Fallon JM: Orthopedic and neurological conditions of pregnancy, Multimedia Presentation, 1990, 1994

Fallon JM: The biomechanical and hormonal considerations of pregnancy as they relate to chiropractic care, Multimedia presentation 1989, 1993, 1994

Fisher AP, Hanna M: Transcutaneous nerve stimulation in meralgia parestetica of pregnancy, British J of Ob Gyn, 94:603, 1987

Font AT, Hankin RS: Pregnancy outcomes after now catastrophic maternal trauma during pregnancy. Obstet Gynecol, 35:912, 1970

Forster JB: Hydrocortisone and the carpal tunnel syndrome, Lancet, 1:456, 1960

Head HB, Welsh JS, Mussey E et.al.: Cyclic sciatica: Report of case with introduction of a new surgical sign. Am Med Assoc, 180:521, 1962

Hamlin E, Lehman RAW: Carpal Tunnel Syndrome, New Engl J Med, 276:849, 1967

Jones MW, Berry K: Chronic relapsing polyneuritis associated with pregnancy, Transactions of the Obstetrical Society of London, 9:12, 1981

Ironside R: Neuritis complicating pregnancy, Proceedings of the Royal Society of Medicine, 32:588, 1939

King G, Ride LT: The relation of vitamin B1 deficiency to pregnancy toxemias. J of Obstet Gynecol of the British Empire, 52:130, 1945

McMullen M: Assessing cervical subluxations in infants under six months of age. Articles on Pediatrics Vol I. International Review of Chiropractic, 1994

McMullen M: Handicapped children and chiropractic care (Part I, II). Articles on Pediatrics Vol 1. International Review of Chiropractic, 1994

O'Connell JEA: Lumbar disc protrusion in pregnancy. J of Neurology, Neurosurgery and Psychiatry, 23:138, 1960

Prineas J: Peripheral nerve changes in thiamine-deficient rats. Archives of Neurology, 23:541, 1970

Sands RX: Bachache of pregnancy: a method of treatment. Obstet Gynecol, 12:670, 1958

Sommerville BW: A study of migraines in pregnancy. Neurology, 22:824, 1972

Strauss MB, McDonald WJ: Polyneuritis of pregnancy: A dietary deficiency disorder. J Amer Med Assoc, 100:1320, 1933

Robinson JR, Pou JW: Bell's Palsy: A predisposition of pregnant women. Archives of Otolaryngology, 95:125, 1972

Romberg MH: Diseases of the Nervous System Vol II, Sydenham Society, London, 1851

Urist MR: Obstetric fracture-dislocation of the pelvis: Report of a case with injury to the lumbosacral trunk and first sacral nerve roots. J Am Med Assoc, 152:127, 1953

Orthopedic/Neurological Conditions

Berg G, Hammar M, Moller-Nielsen J et.al.: Low back pain during pregnancy. Obstet and gynecol, 72:71, 1988

Cohen BA, London RS, Goldstein PJ: Myastenia gravis and preeclampsia. Obstet and Gynecol, 48:35s, 1976

Davis FA: Impairment of repetitive impulse conduction in experimentally demyelinated and pressure injured nerves. J Neurol Neurosurg Psychiatry, 39:443, 1972

Dalessio DJ: Classification and treatment of headache during pregnancy. Clinical Neuropharmocology, 9:121, 1986

Fallon JM: Orthopedic and neurological conditions of pregnancy, Multimedia Presentation, 1990

Fallon JM: The biomechanical and hormonal considerations of pregnancy as they relate to chiropractic care, Multimedia presentation 1989, 1993

Farfan HF: Mechanical Disorders of the Low Back, Lea & Febiger, Philadelphia, 1973

Gelb HGL: Clinical Management of Head, Neck and TMJ Pain and Dysfunction. Saunders, Philadelphia, 1977

Gilliatt RW: The cause of nerve damage in acute compression. Trans Am Neurol Assoc, 99:71,1974

Haldemen S (ed): Modern Developments in the Principles and Practice of Chiropractic, Appleton-Century-Crofts, New York,1980

Haldeman S: Interactions between the somatic and visceral nervous systems. ACA J Chiropractic, 5:57, 1971.

Hammar M, Larsson L, Tegler L: Calcium treatment of leg cramps in pregnancy. Acta Obstetrica et Gynecologia Scandinavica, 60:345, 1981

Homewood AE: The Neurodynamics of the Vertebral Subluxation. Valkyrie Press, St. Petersburg, 1979

Janse JH, Wells BF, et.al: Chiropractic Principles and Technic, National College of Chiropractic, Chicago, 1947

Kopell HP: Help For Your Aching Back, Grosset & Dunlap, New York, 1969

LaBan MM, Perrin JCS, Latimer FR: Pregnancy and the herniated lumbar disc. Archives of Phy. Med and Rehabil. 64:320, 1983

Leach RA: The Chiropractic Theories, Williams & Wilkins, Baltimore, 1986

Lind GAM: Auto-Traction Treatment of Low Back Pain and Sciatica. Linkoping, Sweden, 1974

Lord JW Jr, Rosalie LM: Neurovascular Compression Syndromes of the Upper Extremity. Clin Symp 23:2, 1971

Lowe TW, Weinreb J, Santos-Ramos R et.al.: Magnetic resonance imaging in human pregnancy. Obstet and Gynecol, 66:629, 1985

Lusted LB, Leats TE: Atlas of Roentgenographic Measurement. (2nd ed.) Chicago Yearbook, Chicago, 1967

MacGibbon B, Farfan HF: Are all lumbar spines the same- radiological survey. Spine, 4:258, 1979

Oswald I: Sudden body jerks on falling asleep. Brain, 82:92, 1959

Pacher AR, Steere AC: The triad of neurological manifestations of Lyme disease. Neurology, 35:47, 1986

Palmateer DC: Greater occipital-trigeminal syndrome. J Clin Chiropractic (arch ed.), Winter 1972

Poser S, Poser W: Multiple sclerosis and gestatation. Neurology, 33:1422, 1983

Putti V: New conceptions in the pathogenesis of sciatic pain, Lancet, 2:53, 1927

Rainer GW, Mayer J, Sadler TR, Dirks D: Effects of graded compression on nerve conduction velocity. Arch Surg, 107:719, 1973

Reik L, Steere AC, Bartenhagen NH et. al.: Neurological abnormalities of Lyme disease without erythema chronicum migrans. Amer J of Medicine, 81:73, 1986

Schmorl G, Junghanns H: The Human Spine in Health and Disease (2nd ed.) Grune & Stratton, New York, 1971

Suh CH: Computer Aided Design Mechanisms. University of Colorado, Boulder, 1975

Wall PD, Waxman S, Basbaum AI: Ongoing activity in peripheral nerve: Injury discharge. Exp Neurol, 45:576, 1974

Wright DO, Patel MK: Focal migraine and pregnancy. British Med Journal, 293:1557, 1986

Anatomy & Physiology

Austin CR: Fertilization. Englewood Cliffs, N.J., Prentice-Hall, 1965

Austin CR: Sperm maturation in the male and female genital tracts. In Metz CB.Monray A (eds): Biology of Fertilization, Volume 2, Academic Press, New York, 1985

Braude P, Bolton V, Moore S: Human gene expression first occurs between the four- and eight-cell stages of the preimplantation development. Nature, 332:459, 1988

Braunstein GD, Rasor JL, Engvall E, et.al.: Interrelationships of human chorionic gonadatropin, human placental lactogen and pregnancy-specific glycoprotein throughout normal human gestation. Am J Obstet Gynecol, 138:1205, 1980

Csapo AL, Pulkkinen MO: Indispensability of the human corpus luteum in the maintenance of early pregnancy luteectomy evidence. Obstet Gynecol Surv, 33:69, 1978

Eastman NJ, Hellman LM: Williams Obstetrics, 13th ed. Appleton-Century-Crofts, New York, 1966

Fallon JM: Orthopedic and neurological conditions of pregnancy, Multimedia Presentation, 1990

Fallon JM: The biomechanical and hormonal considerations of pregnancy as they relate to chiropractic care, Multimedia presentation 1989, 1993

Gill TJ III, Immunity and Pregnancy. CRC Crit Rev Immunol, 5:201, 1985

Grant JCB: An Atlas of the Human Body. 7th ed. Williams and Wilkins, Baltimore, 1978

Hearn JP: The embryo-maternal dialogue during early pregnancy in primates. J Reprod Fertil, 76:809, 1986

Hunziker RD, Wegmann TG: Placental immunoregulation. CRC Crit Rev Immunol, 6:245, 1987

Knobil E, Neill J (eds): The Physiology of Reproduction, Raven Press, New York, 1988

Lenton EA, Neal LM, Sulaiman R: Plasma concentrations of human chorionic gonadatropin from the time of implantation until the second week of pregnancy. Fertil Steril, 37:773 1982

Ludwig H, Metzer H, The Human Female Reproductive Tract. A Scanning Electron Microscope Atlas, Springer-Verlag, Heidelberg, 1976

McMullen M: Assessing cervical subluxations in infants under six months of age. Articles on Pediatrics Vol I. International Review of Chiropractic, 1994

Moore KL: The Developing Human, 4th ed. WB Saunders, Philadelphia, 1988

Pauerstein CJ, Hodgson BJ, Kramen MA: The anatomy and physiology of the oviduct. Obstet Gynecol Ann, 3:317 1974

Scott JR,DiSaia PJ, Hammond CB, Spellacy WN. Danforth's Obstetrics and Gynecology 6th ed. J.B. Lippincott Company, Philadelphia, 1990

Sholls HT, Orsini MW, Hitchins DJ: Estrogen synthesis and metabolism in the hamster blastocyst, uterus and liver near the time of implantation. J Steroid Biochemistry, 19:1153 1983

Ulfelder H: Mechanism of pelvic support in women. Am J of Obstet Gynecol, 72:856, 1956

Wynn RM(ed) Cellular Biology of the Uterus, Appleton-Century-Crofts, New York, 1967

6 The Subluxation Complex of Pregnancy

The subluxation is dealt with here as a complex due to its multifaceted etiology. Subluxation in pregnancy is both hormonally and biomechanically induced, and it is important to examine both carefully. It is also important to keep in mind that the subluxation has many effects during pregnancy, only some of which relate to the biomechanics of the spine. While the presence of subluxation is only just beginning to receive the proper acceptance in the medical field, it was described as occurring in the pregnant woman a long time ago. *Gray's Anatomy* states the following:

"During pregnancy the pelvic joints and ligaments are relaxed and capable of more extensive movements. This relationship renders the locking mechanism of the sacroiliac joint less restrictive and permits greater rotation. This change allows alterations in the diameter of the pelvis at childbirth. The less the locking mechanism, the more the strain of weight-bearing falls on the ligaments leading to the frequent occurrence of sacroiliac strain after pregnancy. After childbirth the ligaments become tightened up but in some cases the locking may occur in the position of rotation of the hip bones adopted during pregnancy. This *so-called* **subluxation** of the sacroiliac joint causes pain by the unusual tension which it imposes on the ligaments and the reduction by forceable manipulation may be attempted."

Berg et.al. in their 1988 article *Low Back Pain during Pregnancy* describe how the majority of the low back pain of pregnancy is associated with dysfunction of the SI joints. In an earlier chapter we saw how the SI joints undergo a significant series of changes due to the hormonal and biomechanical stresses.

Alteration of supporting structures

The hormones play a significant role in the alteration of the motor units of the spine. Progesterone decreases smooth muscle tone and this alters the vascular supply to the motor unit as well as the surrounding structures and all of the joints of the body. Estrogen relaxes the joint capsule allowing for more "play" in the joints, including those of the pelvis. This "relaxation" effect is important in that it allows, among many things, for the pelvis to open sufficiently to allow the head and shoulders of the baby to pass through. The hormone relaxin also allows for this to occur.

Subluxation model

Weight gain during pregnancy usually results in an increase of approximately 25-30 lbs. In Chapter 4 we examined weight gain in relation to nutrition. Here we will look at weight gain solely as a function of an increase in lordosis.

In 1947 Dr. Janse Houser and Wells in their definitive work, *Chiropractic Principles and Technic,* proposed a model of lordotic subluxation that I will apply here to pregnancy. In their model they state: "If the head and the chest are thrown too far backward and the weight is thrown upon the articular processes, the inferior articular process will have a tendency to slide backward on the superior articular process of the vertebra below, and in this way will force the latter forward into the intervetebral foramen. (Figures 1 A & B). Such a condition which might be termed a 'physiological lordosis' is seen very commonly in fleshy people, who in order to maintain their balance, lean backward and by doing so throw the lumbar position of the spine forward."

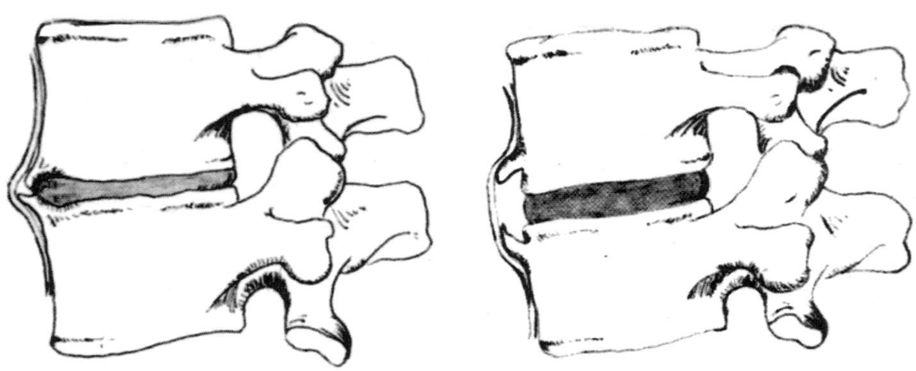

A B

FIGURE 1

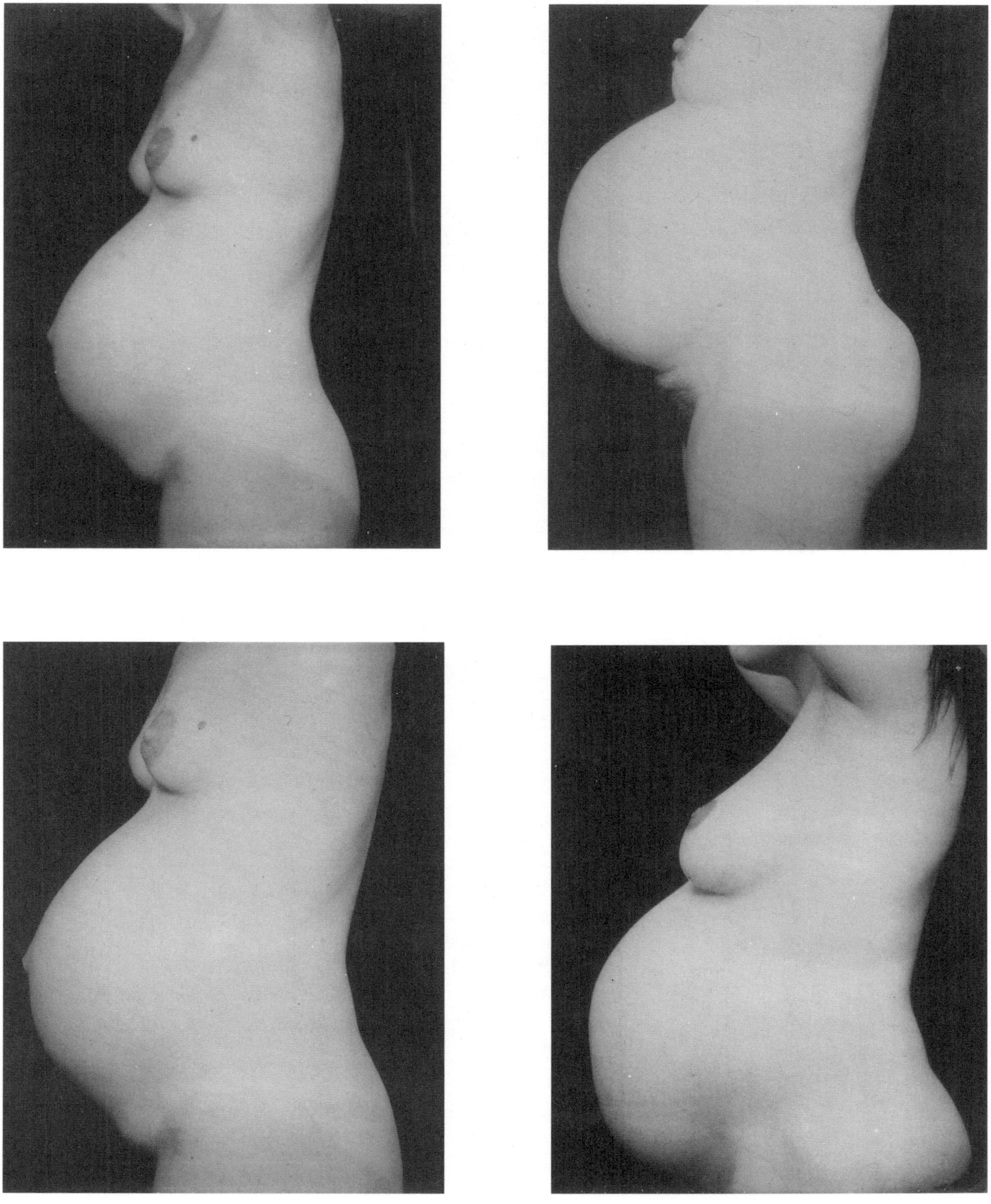

FIGURE 2

These words can simply be applied to the pregnant woman due to her increase in lordosis and is most commonly referred to as the "Pride of Pregnancy." Figure 2 represents some of the lordotic changes that occur during pregnancy. Note in each picture the significant weight distribution in the hips, buttocks, breasts and abdomen.

Other than the obvious changes that occur in the lumbar spine, significant changes occur in other parts of the spine, most noticeably the pelvis. In Chapter 9 we will see different subluxative conditions of the pelvis in pregnancy. Here we will look at the mechanism for subluxation in the pelvis. The following are the varying measurements of the pelvis.

The following demonstrate the different types of pelvises found in the human anatomy. They are characterized in these categories by the shape of the inlet.

Gynecoid

Approximately 50% of women have this type of pelvis (Figure 3). It is the classic female pelvis. It is suited best for childbirth and usually is predisposed to a occiput anterior position of the fetus. It is characterized by a round inlet and a transverse diameter only slightly larger than the anterior posterior diameter. The walls are straight and the sacrum is well curved.

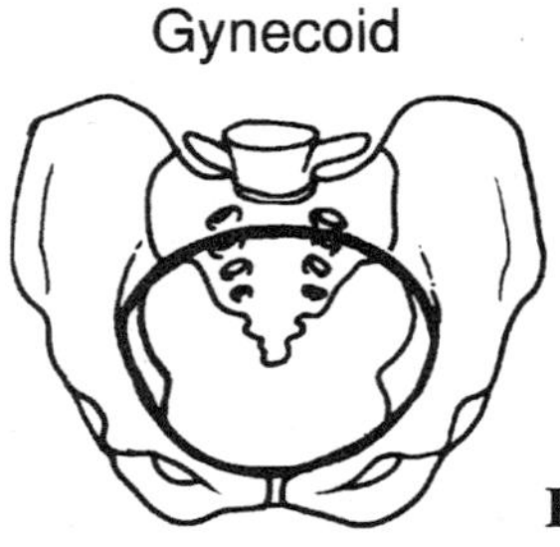

FIGURE 3

Anthropoid

Found in approximately 20% of women it is well suited like the gynecoid pelvis for childbirth. It has straight side walls and an oval inlet. The sacrum is usually posterior in attitude and has a larger anteroposterior than transverse diameter (Figure 4).

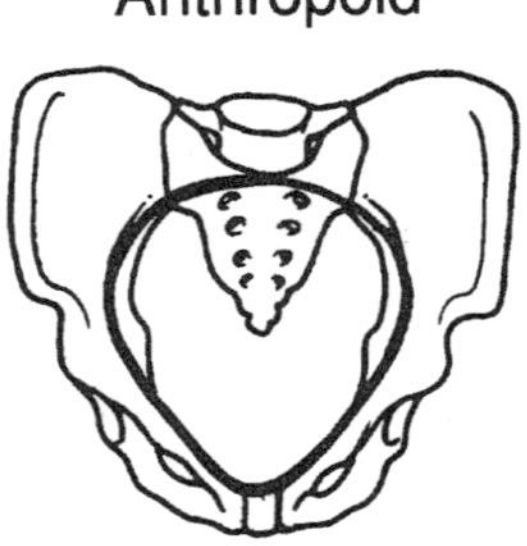

FIGURE 4

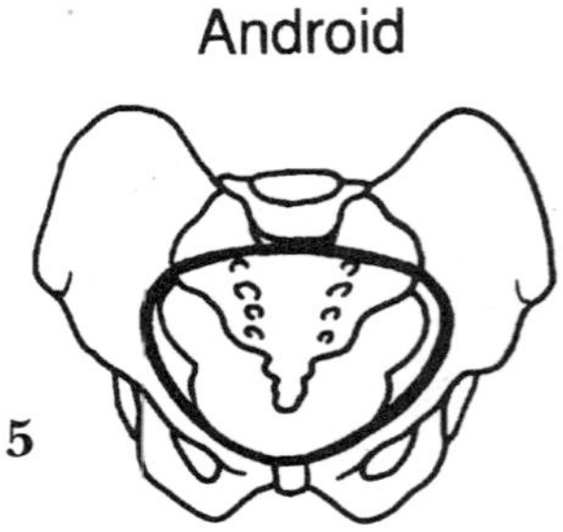

FIGURE 5

Android

This is the typical male pelvis and is found in approximately 30% of women. It is characterized by a triangular inlet and a flat sacrum. As the fetus descends through the pelvis it will have an increasingly difficult time as the outlet narrows (Figure 5).

Platypelloid

Also known as a flat pelvis it is a flattened version of the gynecoid pelvis. The inlet is somewhat kidney shaped and presents difficulty for the fetus at the brim. Once the fetus descends below the brim it has less trouble moving through. It is found in approximately 3% of women (Figure 6).

Platypelloid

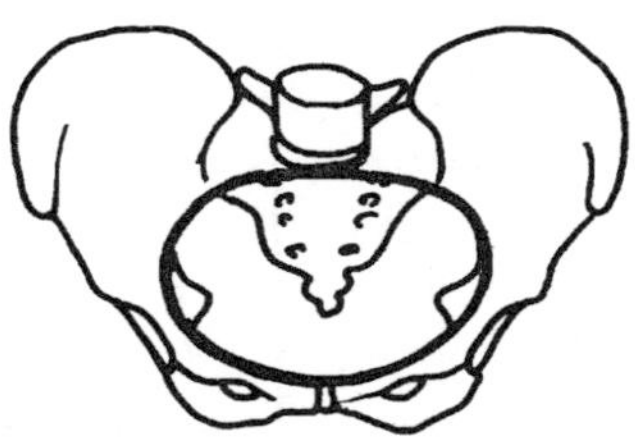

FIGURE 6

When considering the pelvis and the birth process, it is important to discuss engagement and pelvic stations. Pelvic *engagement* occurs when the largest diameter of the fetal presenting part enters and passes through the pelvic inlet. The *station* is the level above or below the level of the ischial spines. 0 is assigned to the level of the ishial spine. Each centimeter above is designated as a (-) and each centimeter below as a (+) with the range being from -3 to +3. When the fetal head is above -3 the head is said to be *floating* and when it presents below the level of the inlet intermittently, it is said to be *dipping*.

Subluxations of the pelvis can occur in three separate places. Each sacroiliac joint and the symphysis pubis joint are susceptible to subluxation and do readily occur in pregnancy. In addition to the influences of the hormones, the weight gain, and the alterations of the supporting structures on each of the joint components of the pelvis, different types of pelvises exert differing stresses during pregnancy. Both the gynecoid and anthropoid pelvises accommodate the head of the fetus well and subject that head to equal force as the fetus descends during birth. The android pelvis has a large opening superiorly and narrows inferiorly. As the fetal head engages in the pelvis and continues its descent it will tend to cause Superior/Inferior

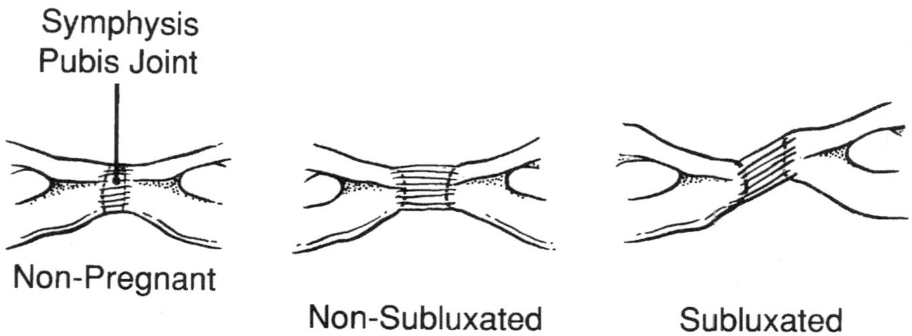

FIGURE 7

Sl subluxation due to the narrowing effect of the pelvis and the gravitational pushing of the fetus. In contrast, the flat pelvis or platypelloid pelvis is narrow superiorly and widens inferiorly. This type of pelvis will tend to subluxate at the symphysis pubis joint. (Figure 7)

There are other factors which come to bear on the pelvis and the type of subluxations that occur. Some of the considerations are: number of pregnancies, status of the pelvic musculature, lifestyle, levels of exercise, and past trauma to the pelvis. Women who are multiparous have the greatest tendency towards pelvic subluxation. With each successive pregnancy the pelvic musculature and ligamentous structures become stretched and predispose the pelvis to subluxation. In that same vain, it becomes easier to correct subluxation in these women. Often times women who subluxate as a function of successive pregnancies will subluxate in the same way during each pregnancy.

Thoracic and cervical subluxation tend to follow a more normal course of cause and effect due to the presence of the hormones of pregnancy, and the pregnancy stresses on the body. The weight gain and alteration of supporting structures will play a part in the subluxations of the cervical and thoracic spine. Chapter 5 describes in detail the varying conditions of the thoracic and cervical spine associated with subluxation and pregnancy. Thoracic subluxation will be first to appear during pregnancy due to the changes that occur in the flattening of the rib cage that appears early in pregnancy. Intercostal neuralgia is the most common subluxative condition seen early in pregnancy due to this anatomical change. Exaggeration of the kyphotic curve will also induce subluxative changes in the thoracic spine. Since the majority of the changes that occur in the pregnancy state occur in the lower half of the woman's body, the changes that occur in the cervical spine are secondary to the changes that occur elsewhere in the spine. It is important to note that the hormonal changes and the weight gain will also produce some change in the cervical spine.

Correction of subluxation during pregnancy is a simple task when compared to the non-pregnant state. While the hormonal changes affect the musculature and ligamentous structures often times producing subluxation, in the same way those changes allow for ease of correction of the subluxation. One of the most frequently asked questions is, "Can adjustments in pregnancy produce miscarriage?" The answer to that question is definitely NO. The amount of thrust needed to correct a subluxation during pregnancy is minimal compared to that needed in the non-pregnant state. One must keep in mind that very often miscarriage is the body's way of ridding itself of a defective fetus. If the woman's body is in a subluxated state, its ability to perceive that defect may be impaired. If an adjustment restores that intelligence to the body, then miscarriage may occur. All pregnant women should be made aware of that possibility prior to receiving treatment. Simple adjusting cannot harm the fetus nor will it produce spontaneous abortion when not indicated for other reasons.

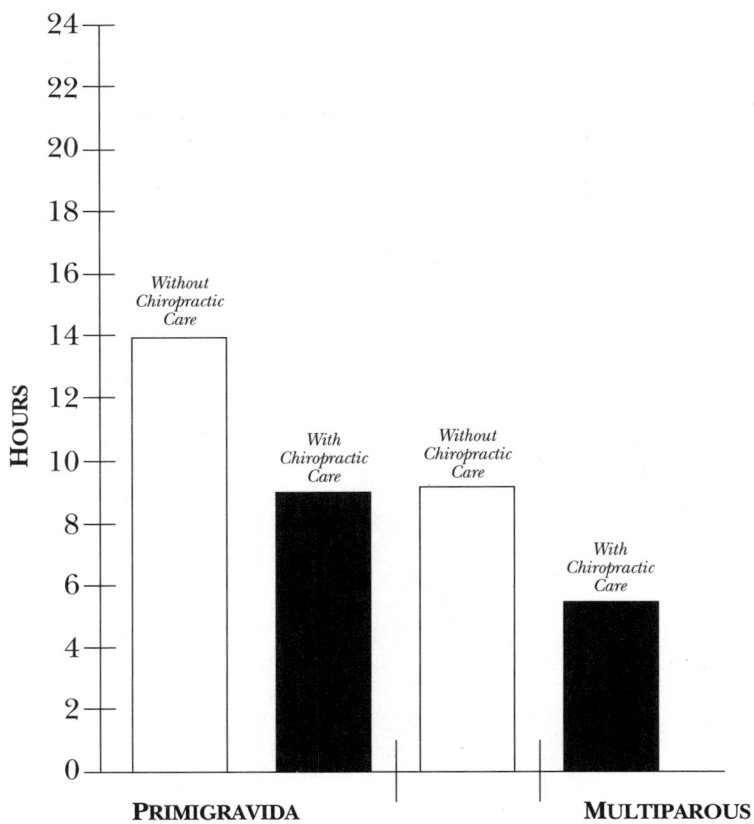

FIGURE 8

Effect of chiropractic adjustments on labor

Statistics from the author's office have demonstrated that chiropractic adjustments effectively reduce the average amount of time spent in labor. Forty-seven primagravida and 67 multiparous women were compared as to their mean duration of labor (Figure 8). Only women who were seen beginning in the first to tenth week throughout their pregnancy were used for comparison purposes. Any woman who was seen specifically for a condition that presented during the last trimester was excluded from the study. The term "labor" was defined as the onset of timeable rhythmic contractions. (It should be noted that this was not a controlled study but statistics taken from the author's office files. It is time however for controlled studies to be undertaken on this subject.)

The generally accepted mean labor times are 12-14 hours for the primigravida, and 8-10 hours in the multiparous. These numbers are quite conservative and the actual labor can sometimes last much longer.

The results of the author's case history work are depicted in Figure 8. It is easy to see that with all else being equal the mean labor time with chiropractic care is reduced by nearly 25% compared to the generally accepted mean labor time. In the multiparous woman, the reduction was 33%.

Technique

Any number of chiropractic techniques can be used effectively with the pregnant woman. It is important for the chiropractor to know that the types of changes that can occur during pregnancy can be as gross as a luxation of the symphysis pubis and a technique that can correct

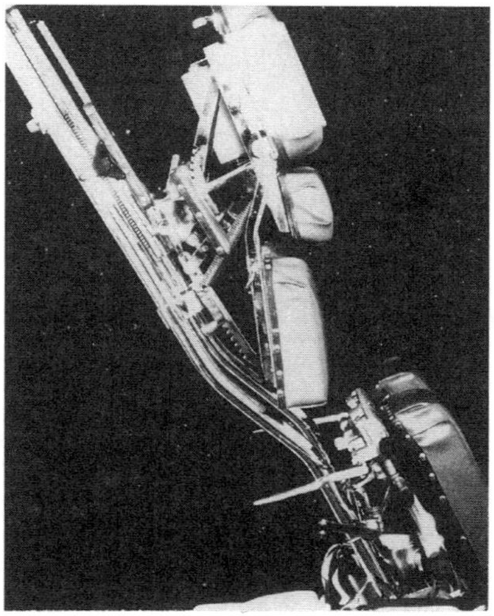

HI-LO TABLE

FIGURE 9

that type of misalignment should be part of the repertoire of each chiropractor. All of the changes that the pregnant woman undergoes is on the gross rather than subtle level. This does not preclude the fact that many subtle changes do occur and must be addressed, but the majority of subluxative changes occur on that gross level.

One of the most common discomforts and complaints that the women have during pregnancy is their inability to lie prone. The chiropractic office is often the only place where a woman can lie flat and be comfortable. The hi-lo with the abdominal cushion forward allows for the pregnant belly to lie flat and to have the exaggerated lordosis corrected.

Cervical spine

Correction of cervical subluxation can be handled in the same fashion that the doctor is accustomed to in the non-pregnant patient. No change needs to occur, only special attention given to the laxity of ligamentous structure.

Thoracic spine

Early changes that occur in the thoracic spine call for early treatment. The changes in the respiratory system and the flattening of the rib cage to accommodate for the increased inspiratory and expiratory volumes change the structure of the entire rib cage. Movement of the thoracic vertebra may need to be employed as well as adjustment of the ribs themselves. Rib head displacement is quite common.

Lumbar spine

Lumbar subluxation and its theories have been examined elsewhere in this chapter and in Chapter 5, but it is important to consider the direction of subluxation at the lumbar vertebrae. In the Janse Howser et.al model of posterior slippage due to the anterior weight of the pregnancy, it is clear that spinous imbrication is a distinct possibility and must be accommodated for in the adjusting procedure. Subluxation of the lumbar vertebrae occur in the same fashion as in the non-pregnant patient with the exception that the misalignment will be far more exaggerated due to the lumbar lordosis. Traditional side posture, Diversified or Knee Chest moves are completely appropriate for the lumbar spine. As has been pointed out before, minimal thrusting is necessary to make a correction during pregnancy. Activator and other techniques can also be employed.

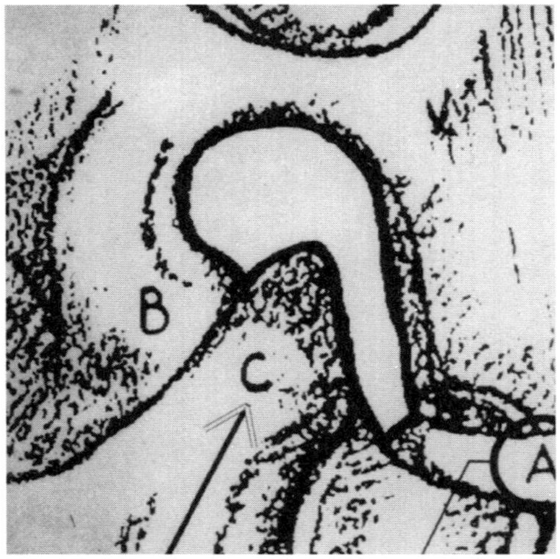

SUBLUXATION COMPLEX OF PREGNANCY

FIGURE 10

Pelvis

Earlier in this chapter the pelvis was examined in detail as to their types and the problems associated with birth. Unlike the other sections of the spine, the pelvis will subluxate in the pregnant woman in configurations unfamiliar to the chiropractor who does not as a rule treat pregnant women. The two SI joints and the SP joint move in a total of 13 different ways. Each in its regular plane of motion and in addition a separation can occur in each location. When the possible combinations of these movements are examined the possibilities are limitless, and require a special eye to the changes that occur here. Special improvisation of adjustive techniques is needed.

Treatment protocol

One of the most frequently asked questions is how often should a pregnant woman be adjusted? That question is difficult to answer and can vary from patient to patient. With experience one will be able to assess the changes in the body that occur duirng pregnancy and set

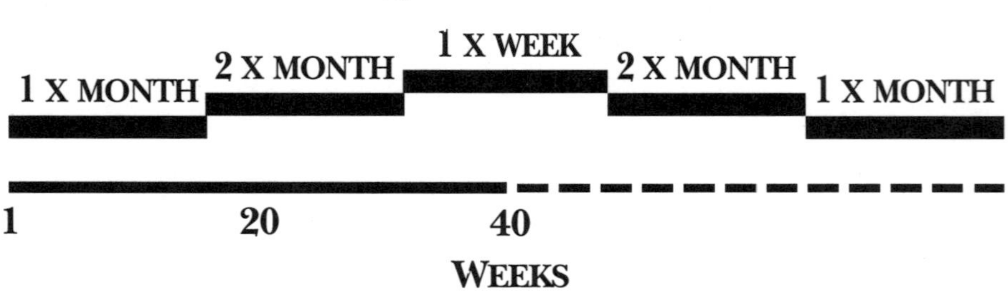

up the treatment protocol accordingly. The diagram on the previous page most closely depicts the necessity of chiropractic adjustments during pregnancy.

We see that these visits are spaced in much the same as the visits to the obstetrician/midwife. With each successive change that occurs in the pregnant woman, it is important to check her spine to assess the subluxative changes. In the last trimester with the great increase in size of the fetus, the woman's spine will undergo significant changes that warrant frequent visits to the chiropractor. ■

REFERENCES

Orthopedic/Neurological Conditions

Berg G, Hammar M, Moller-Nielsen J et.al.: Low back pain during pregnancy. Obstet and gynecol, 72:71, 1988

Cohen BA, London RS, Goldstein PJ: Myastenia gravis and preeclampsia. Obstet and Gynecol, 48:35s, 1976

Davis FA: Impairment of repetitive impulse conduction in experimentally demyelinated and pressure injured nerves. J Neurol Neurosurg, Psychiatry, 39:443, 1972

Dalessio DJ: Classification and treatment of headache during pregnancy. Clinical Neuropharmocology, 9:121, 1986

Fallon JM: Orthopedic and neurological conditions of pregnancy, Multimedia Presentation, 1990

Fallon JM: The biomechanical and hormonal considerations of pregnancy as they relate to chiropractic care, Multimedia presentation 1989, 1993

Farfan HF: Mechanical Disorders of the Low Back, Lea & Febiger, Philadelphia, 1973

Gelb HGL: Clinical Management of Head, Neck and TMJ Pain and Dysfunction. Saunders, Philadelphia, 1977

Gilliatt RW: The cause of nerve damage in acute compression. Trans Am Neurol Assoc, 99:71, 1974

Haldemen S (ed): Modern Developments in the Principles and Practice of Chiropractic, Appleton-Century-Crofts, New York, 1980

Haldeman S: Interactions between the somatic and visceral nervous systems. ACA J Chiropractic, 5:57, 1971

Hammar M, Larsson L, Tegler L: Calcium treatment of leg cramps in pregnancy. Acta Obstetrica et Gynecologia Scandinavica, 60:345, 1981

Homewood AE: The Neurodynamics of the Vertebral Subluxation. Valkyrie Press, St. Petersburg, 1979

Janse JH, Wells BF, et.al: Chiropractic Principles and Technic, National College of Chiropractic, Chicago, 1947

Kopell HP: Help For Your Aching Back, Grosset & Dunlap, New York,1969

LaBan MM, Perrin JCS, Latimer FR: Pregnancy and the herniated lumbar disc. Archives of Phy. Med and Rehabil. 64:320, 1983

Leach RA: The Chiropractic Theories, Williams & Wilkins, Baltimore, 1986

Lind GAM: Auto-Traction Treatment of Low Back Pain and Sciatica. Linkoping, Sweden, 1974

Lord JW Jr, Rosalie LM: Neurovascular Compression Syndromes of the Upper Extremity. Clin Symp, 23:2, 1971

Lowe TW, Weinreb J, Santos-Ramos R et.al.:Magnetic resonance imaging in human pregnancy. Obstet and Gynecol, 66:629, 1985

Lusted LB, Leats TE: Atlas of Roentgenographic Measurement. (2nd ed.) Chicago Yearbook, Chicago, 1967

MacGibbon B, Farfan HF: Are all lumbar spines the same- radiological survey. Spine, 4:258, 1979

Oswald I: Sudden body jerks on falling asleep. Brain, 82:92, 1959

Pacher AR, Steere AC: The triad of neurological manifestations of Lyme disease. Neurology, 35:47, 1986

Palmateer DC: Greater occipital-trigeminal syndrome. J Clin Chiropractic (arch ed.), Winter 1972

Poser S, Poser W: Multiple sclerosis and gestatation. Neurology, 33:1422, 1983

Putti V: New conceptions in the pathogenesis of sciatic pain. Lancet, 2:53, 1927

Rainer GW, Mayer J, Sadler TR, Dirks D: Effects of graded compression on nerve conduction velocity. Arch Surg, 107:719, 1973

Reik L, Steere AC,Bartenhagen NH et. al.: Neurological abnormalities of Lyme disease without erythema chronicum migrans. Amer J of Medicine, 81:73, 1986

Schmorl G, Junghanns H: The Human Spine in Health and Disease (2nd ed.) Grune & Stratton, New York, 1971

Suh CH: Computer Aided Design Mechanisms. University of Colorado, Boulder 1975

Wall PD, Waxman S, Basbaum AI: Ongoing activity in peripheral nerve: Injury discharge. Exp Neurol, 45:576, 1974

Wright DO,Patel MK: Focal migraine and pregnancy. British Med Journal 293:1557, 1986

Systemic Changes During Pregnancy

Anderson LL: Regulation of relaxin secretion and it's role in pregnancy. Adv Exp Med Biol, 219:421, 1987

Baird JD: Some aspects of the metabolic and hormonal adaptation to pregnancy. Acta Endocrinol (suppl) (Copenh), 277:11, 1986

Brody SA, Ueland K (eds): Endocrine Disorders in Pregnancy, Appleton & Lange, Norwalk, 1989

Chesley LC, Sibai BM: Blood pressure in the midtrimester and future pre-eclampsia. Am J Obstet Gynecol 157:1258, 1987

Davison JM: Kidney function in pregnant women. Am J Kidney Dis 9:265, 1987

DeSwiet M: The respiratory system. In Hytten FE, Chamberlain G(eds): Clinical Physiology in Obstetrics, 2nd ed. Blackwell, Oxford, 1991

Douvas SG, Meeks GR, Phillips JC, et.al.: Liver disease in pregnancy. Obstet Gynecol Surv, 38:531, 1983

Easterling TR, Schumucker BC, Benedetti TJ: The haemodynamic effects of orthostatic stress during pregnancy. Obstet Gynecol, 72:550, 1988

Fallon JM: Orthopedic and neurological conditions of pregnancy, Multimedia Presentation, 1990

Fallon JM: The biomechanical and hormonal considerations of pregnancy as they relate to chiropractic care, Multimedia presentation 1989, 1993

Gant NF, Whalley PJ, Everett RB, et.al.: Control of vascular reactivity in pregnancy. Am. J. Kidney Disease, 9:303, 1987

Grant JCB: An Atlas of the Human Body. 7th ed. Baltimore, Williams and Wilkins, 1978

Klein EA: Urologic problems in pregnancy: A review. Obstet Gyecol Surv, 39:605, 1984

Lind T: Metabolic changes in pregnancy relevant to diabetes mellitus. Postgrad Med J, 55:353, 1979

Macfie AG, Magides AP, et. al.: Gastric emptying in pregnancy. Br J Anaesth, 67:54, 1991

Metcalfe J, McAnulty JH, Ueland K: Burwell and Metcalfe's Heart Disease in Pregnancy: Physiology and Management. Little, Brown, Boston, 1986

Milne JS, Howie AD, Pack AI: Dyspnoea during normal pregnancy. Br. J Obstet Gynaecol, 85:260, 1978

Pritchard JA, Scott DE: Iron stores of normal adults and their replenishment with oral iron therapy. J Amer Med Assoc, 190:897, 1964

Smout CFV, Jacoby F, Lillie EW: Gynecological and Obstetrical Anatomy. Williams and Wilkins, Baltimore, 1969

Anatomy & Physiology

Austin CR: Fertilization. Prentice-Hall, Englewood Cliffs, N.J., 1965

Austin CR: Sperm maturation in the male and female genital tracts. In Metz CB. Monray A (eds): Biology of Fertilization, Volume 2, Academic Press, New York, 1985

Braude P, Bolton V, Moore S: Human gene expression first occurs between the four- and eight-cell stages of the preimplantation development. Nature, 332:459, 1988

Braunstein GD, Rasor JL, Engvall E, et.al.: Interrelationships of human chorionic gonadatropin, human placental lactogen and pregnancy-specific glycoprotein throughout normal human gestation. Am J Obstet Gynecol, 138:1205, 1980

Csapo AL, Pulkkinen MO: Indispensability of the human corpus luteum in the maintenance of early pregnancy luteectomy evidence. Obstet Gynecol Surv, 33:69, 1978

Eastman NJ, Hellman LM: Williams Obstetrics, 13th ed. Appleton-Century-Crofts, New York, 1966

Fallon JM: Orthopedic and neurological conditions of pregnancy, Multimedia Presentation, 1990

Fallon JM: The biomechanical and hormonal considerations of pregnancy as they relate to chiropractic care, Multimedia presentation 1989, 1993

Gill TJ III, Immunity and Pregnancy. CRC Crit Rev Immunol, 5:201, 1985

Grant JCB: An Atlas of the Human Body. 7th ed. Williams and Wilkins, Baltimore, 1978

Hearn JP: The embryo-maternal dialogue during early pregnancy in primates. J Reprod Fertil, 76:809, 1986

Hunziker RD, Wegmann TG, Placental immunoregulation. CRC Crit Rev Immunol, 6:245, 1987

Knobil E, Neill J (eds): The Physiology of Reproduction, Raven Press, New York, 1988

Lenton EA, Neal LM, Sulaiman R: Plasma concentrations of human chorionic gonadatropin from the time of implantation until the second week of pregnancy. Fertil Steril, 37:773, 1982

Ludwig H, Metzer H: The Human Female Reproductive Tract. A Scanning Electron Microscope Atlas, Springer-Verlag, Heidelberg, 1976

McMullen M: Assessing cervical subluxations in infants under six months of age. Articles on Pediatrics Vol I. International Review of Chiropractic, 1994

Moore KL: The Developing Human, 4th ed. WB Saunders, Philadelphia, 1988

Pauerstein CJ, Hodgson BJ, Kramen MA: The anatomy and physiology of the oviduct. Obstet Gynecol Ann, 3:317, 1974

Scott JR, DiSaia PJ, Hammond CB, Spellacy WN. Danforth's Obstetrics and Gynecology 6th ed. J.B. Lippincott Company, Philadelphia, 1990

Sholls HT, Orsini MW, Hitchins DJ: Estrogen synthesis and metabolism in the hamster blastocyst, uterus and liver near the time of implantation. J Steroid Biochemistry, 19:1153, 1983

Ulfelder H: Mechanism of pelvic support in women. Am J of Obstet Gynecol, 72:856, 1956

Wynn RM(ed) Cellular Biology of the Uterus, Appleton-Century-Crofts, New York, 1967

Neuromuscular Skeletal System

Adour KK: The bell tolls for decompression? New England Journal of Medicine, 292:748, 1975

Aminoff MJ: Neurological disorders and pregnancy. Am J Obstet Gynecol, 132:325, 1978

Bell C: The Nervous System of the Human Body. Longman Rees, Orme, Brown, and Green, London, 1830

Berg G, Hammer M, Moller-Nielson J, et al: Low back pain during pregnancy. Obstetrics and Gynecology, 72:71

Berkwitz NJ and Lufkin NH: Toxic neuronitis of pregnancy: A clinicopathological report. Surgery, Gynecology and Obstetrics, 54:743, 1932

Benson RC, Inman VT: Brachialgia statica dysesthetica in pregnancy. Western Journal of Surgery, 64:115, 1956

Brown JT and McDougall A: Traumatic maternal birth palsy, Journal of Obstetrics and Gynecology of the British Empire, 64:431

Cole JT: Maternal obstetric paralysis, American Journal of Obstetrics and Gynecology, 52:386

Ecker AD and Woltman HW: Meralgia Parestetica: A report of one hundred and fifty cases. J Amer Med Assoc, 110:1650, 1938

Eckman-Ordeberg G, Salgeback S, Ordeberg G: Carpal Tunnel Syndrome in pregnancy: A prospective study. Acta Obstet Gynecol Scand, 66:233, 1987

Fallon JM: Orthopedic and neurological conditions of pregnancy and chiropractic management of care. Articles on Pediatrics Vol II, International review of Chiropractic, 1994

Fallon JM: Orthopedic and neurological conditions of pregnancy, Multimedia Presentation, 1990, 1994

Fallon JM: The biomechanical and hormonal considerations of pregnancy as they relate to chiropractic care, Multimedia presentation 1989, 1993, 1994

Fisher AP, Hanna M: Transcutaneous nerve stimulation in meralgia parestetica of pregnancy, British J of Ob Gyn, 94:603, 1987

Font AT, Hankin RS: Pregnancy outcomes after now catastrophic maternal trauma during pregnancy. Obstet Gynecol, 35:912, 1970

Forster JB: Hydrocortisone and the carpal tunnel syndrome, Lancet, 1:456, 1960

Head HB, Welsh JS, Mussey E et al: Cyclic sciatica: Report of case with introduction of a new surgical sign. J Amer Med Assoc, 180:521, 1962

Hamlin E, Lehman RAW: Carpal Tunnel Syndrome, New Engl J Med, 276:849, 1967

Jones MW, Berry K: Chronic relapsing polyneuritis associated with pregnancy, Transactions of the Obstetrical Society of London, 9:12, 1981

Ironside R: Neuritis complicating pregnancy, Proceedings of the Royal Society of Medicine, 32:588, 1939

King G, Ride LT: The relation of vitamin B1 deficiency to pregnancy toxemias. J of Obstet Gynecol of the British Empire, 52:130, 1945

McMullen M: Assessing cervical subluxations in infants under six months of age. Articles on Pediatrics Vol I. International Review of Chiropractic, 1994

McMullen M: Handicapped children and chiropractic care (Part I & II). Articles on Pediatrics Vol 1. International Review of Chiropractic, 1994

O'Connell JEA: Lumbar disc protrusion in pregnancy. J of Neurology, Neurosurgery and Psychiatry, 23:138, 1960

Prineas J: Peripheral nerve changes in thiamine-deficient rats. Archives of Neurology, 23:541, 1970

Sands RX: Bachache of pregnancy: A method of treatment. Obstet Gynecol, 12:670, 1958

Sommerville BW: A study of migraines in pregnancy. Neurology, 22:824, 1972

Strauss MB, McDonald WJ: Polyneuritis of pregnancy: A dietary deficiency disorder. J Amer Med Assoc, 100:1320, 1933

Robinson JR, Pou JW: Bell's Palsy: A predisposition of pregnant women. Archives of Otolaryngology, 95:125, 1972

Romberg MH: Diseases of the Nervous System Vol II, Sydenham Society, London, 1851

Urist MR: Obstetric fracture-dislocation of the pelvis: Report of a case with injury to the lumbosacral trunk and first sacral nerve roots. J Amer Med Assoc, 152:127, 1953

Adjusting the Pregnant Woman

DeBoer KF, Harmon RO, Savoie, Tuttle CD: Inter and intra-examiner reliability of leg length differential measurement: a preliminary study. J Manip Physiolog Ther, 6:61, 1983

Fallon JM: Chiropractic and pregnancy, Articles on Pediatrics Vol I, International Review of Chiropractic, 1994

Fallon JM: Orthopedic and neurological conditions of pregnancy, Multimedia Presentation, 1990

Fallon JM: Orthopedic and neurological conditions of pregnancy and chiropractic management of care, Articles on Pediatrics Vol II, International Review of Chiropractic, 1994

Fallon JM: The Biomechanical and hormonal considerations of pregnancy as they relate to chiropractic care. Multimedia presentation 1989, 1993

Finneson BE (ed): Low Back Pain. Lippincott, Philadelphia, 1980

Grostic J: Some observations on computer-aided x-ray analysis. Int Rev Chiro 33:38, 1979

Haldeman S: Spinal Manipulative Therapy. Clin Orthop, 179:62, 1983

Hamlin E, Lehman RAW: Carpal Tunnel Syndrome, New Engl J Med, 276:849, 1967

Ironside R: Neuritis complicating pregnancy, Proceedings of the Royal Society of Medicine, 32:588, 1939

Palmer DD: The Science, Art and Philosophy of Chiropractic, Portland Printing House, Portland, 1910

Palmer MH: Chiropractic Anatomy Vol IX, Palmer College of Chiropractic, Davenport, 1929

Ulfelder H: Mechanism of pelvic support in women. Am J of Obstet Gynecol, 72:856, 1956

7 Birth Injuries & Subluxation of the Newborn

As we have seen in other parts of this text, the birth process can have a significant effect on the life of the child. One of the most important aspects of the study of pregnancy is the outcome of the birth process and the possible subluxative effects on the newborn. It is important for the chiropractor to be able to determine the subluxative changes that occur in the newborn and there is no better way to do so than to use the McMullen Reverse Fencer Reflex. Discovered and developed by Dr. Maxine McMullen, one of the leading chiropractic practitioners and educators in the field of pregnancy and pediatrics, it is a normal variation of one of the infantile automatisms, the Fencer Reflex. The Fencer response/ Tonic Neck Reflex is elicited at birth with the strength most noticeable during the second and third month of life and disappearing by the sixth month of life. In the straight Fencer reflex the supine infant's head is turned to one side with the infant responding with extension of limbs on the ipsilateral side and the flexion of the limbs on the contralateral side. As with other infantile automatisms this is a protective mechanism.

To elicit the Reverse Fencer/McMullen Response, the infant is gently placed upside down with the examiner first bracing the ankles of the child and lifting them up. The legs are elevated over the buttocks and the buttocks lifted over the torso, until the child is free-hanging from the ankles. This maneuver may elicit a Moro/Startle response but most often the child will be pleased to be in this position (Figure 1). If an extreme arching is noted, it may demonstrate a meningeal irritation, and distress may be noted. If pelvic locking or any type of extreme discomfort is noted the child should be evaluated for subluxation or luxation.

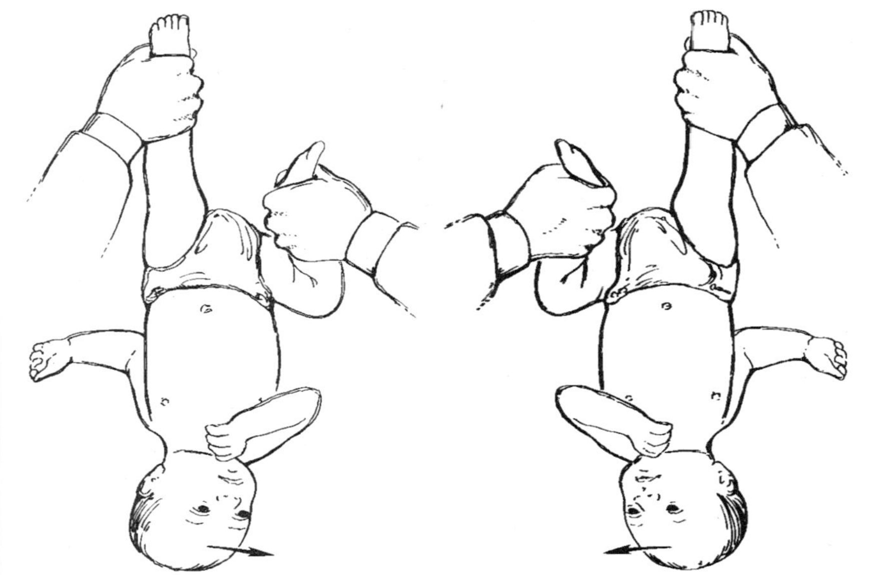

Illustration reprinted with permission from the International Review of Chiropractic, March/April 1990. Illustrator: Terese Winslow.

REVERSE FENCER

FIGURE 1

Once the child is comfortably hanging and one of the legs is flexed, a rotation of the head should occur toward the side of the flexed leg. This is the opposite of what is observed in the supine child where the neck turns toward the extended leg. This movement in the hanging position should be free and easy as long as the child is subluxation free in the upper cervical area. If there is subluxation present in the upper cervical area (atlas/axis/occiput) there will be some discomfort to the head turning mechanism and the child will override the reflexive response and turn the head again to the midline. Upon reaching the midline the reflexive mechanism again begins, the child turns its head to the flexed leg side and being irritated, will again override the response and find itself returning the head position to the midline. This will elicit what Dr. McMullen has referred to as a "twitching" effect and is pathagnomonic of upper cervical subluxation. The process is repeated on the other side, noting any "twitching" and the child is returned to the supine position.

Dr. McMullen goes on to describe a further evaluation to determine the exact subluxation and the differentiation of atlas/axis subluxation vs. atlas/occiput subluxation. The examiner will then place constant pressure by pushing the femur head into the acetabulum on each side, while observing the degree of resistance on each side. Normally the pressure should be equal and firm. When one side appears to be soft or "mushy," that side is thought to be the side of atlas laterality. This "check" is akin to the adult leg check and works on much the same principle. In the absence of a difference on either side, the subluxation is most likely to be that of the occiput. These findings can be confirmed by motion and static palpation.

One of the most commonly asked questions is "how do I feel for subluxation in the newborn when unaccustomed to working with children of that age?" This check will standardize care for the newborn. A simple adjustment of the practitioner's choice can be performed. The atlas and occiput are not completely fused and therefore require simple gentle adjustments. The atlas can take a simple toggle like adjustment while in the arms of the practitioner. A postcheck can be performed once an adjustment is delivered to see if the subluxation has been corrected.

Infantile automatism

One of the best ways the chiropractor can determine the overall neurological health of the newborn is to perform a series of tests which can elicit the infantile automatisms. Some of these automatisms are abnormal reflexes which when present in the adult signal severe neurological impairment, usually of the upper motor neuron lesion variety. The newborn possesses an immature nervous system which begins to mature by the time the child reaches the age of 6 months. These responses often disappear by that time.

The absence of these responses in the newborn signals the possibility of some level of brain damage. Damage of that nature of course can not be based solely on the absence of these responses but they give the chiropractor a quick overall assessment of the neurological health of the child.

Some of the automatisms are as follows:

Blink

Stimulus– shine light in eyes
Response– close eyelids
Duration– 8 months – 1 yr.
Indications– if absent, blindness or eyelid malfunction

Rooting

Stimulus– stroke baby's cheek
Response– baby moves head to side of stroking (stroking resembles the side of the mother's breast)
Duration– 34 months
Indications– if absent can be severe neurological problem (possible upper motor neuron – CNS problem)

Sucking
Stimulus– give child a finger or nipple
Response– The child should begin to suck
Duration– 3-4 months
Indications– if absent possible UMN problem

Moro (Startle)
Stimulus– clap hands or make a loud noise
Response– extension of extremities and opening of the eyes, with rapid following flexion
Duration– 4 months
Indications– its presence beyond 4 – 5 months, neurological
absence altogether– also neurological
assymetrical– possible injury or fracture

Tonic Neck (Fencer)
Stimulus– baby placed supine and head turned to one side
Response– extension of extremities on side of head turn
Duration– 4 – 6 months
Indications– persistence beyond 6 months – poss neurological

Galant
Stimulus – baby face down supported by examiner's arm, examiner's fingers are run paravertebrally from the occiput to the sacrum
Response– buttock torques toward the stimulated side
Duration– 3 – 4 months
Indications– absence or reduction, neurological ranging from damage to paralysis

Perez
Stimulus– baby face down supported by the examiner's arm run fingers over the spinous processes from the sacrum to the occiput
Response– extension of the head, bringing knees to chest, urination
Duration– 24 months
Indications– severe neurological deficit/cerebral dysfunction

Grasp
Stimulus– place examiner's finger in the baby's hand
Response– fingers curl to the stimulus
Duration– 3 – 6 months
Indications– cerebral insult when persistent

Babinski

Stimulus– stroke the sole of the foot medial to lateral and side to side

Response– toes spread out and the great toe dorsiflexes

Duration– 16 – 24 months

Indications– beyond 2 years, neurological defect

Steppage (Placing)

Stimulus– with baby help upright the dirsum of the foot touches the undersurface of the table

Response– places foot on top of table

Duration– variable 2 – 4 months

Indications– absence, poss neurological

It is important to understand that the immaturity of the nervous system is a normal phenomena, and the presence of these responses is normal in the child under the age of 6 months.

Birth Injuries

Abnormal moulding of the cranial bones

As the fetus descends through the birth canal there is a normal moulding of the cranial bones where the anterior parietals overlap the posterior parietals and both parietals overlap the occiput and frontal bones. When the birth involves a malposition, it may result in subluxation of the cranial bones.

Damage to the brachial plexus

The Brachial Plexus can be damaged by lateral flexion to the neck during vertex or breech birth (Figure 2).

1) Erb's Palsy - damage to C5, C6 and is the most common type of problem in this area and will result in a Waiter's Tip deformity (Figure 2).
2) Klumpke's Palsy - Damage to C8, T1 resulting in wrist drop and hand paralysis
3) Horner's Syndrome - interruption of the sympathetic supply to T1 resulting in ptosis, exophthalmosis and meiosis of the eye

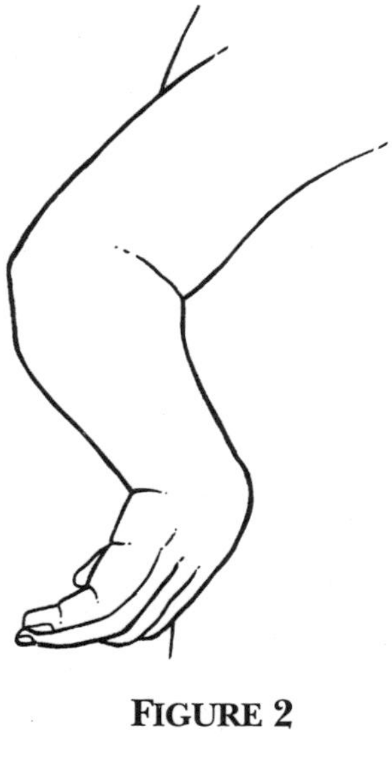

FIGURE 2

Facial paralysis

Results from paralysis of the facial nerve as it exits the stylomastoid foramen. It is most often caused by the use of forceps (Figure 3).

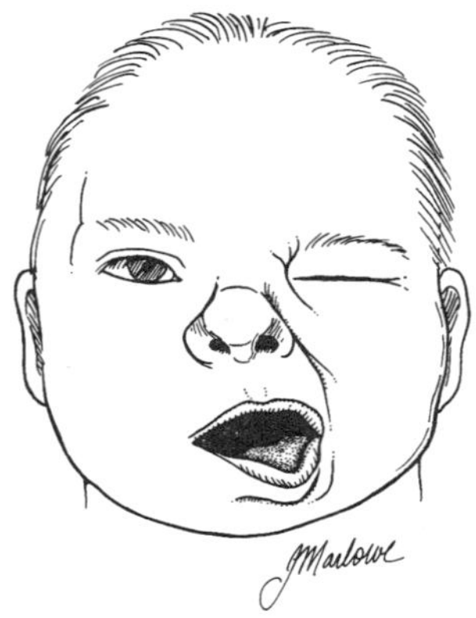

FACIAL PARALYSIS

FIGURE 3

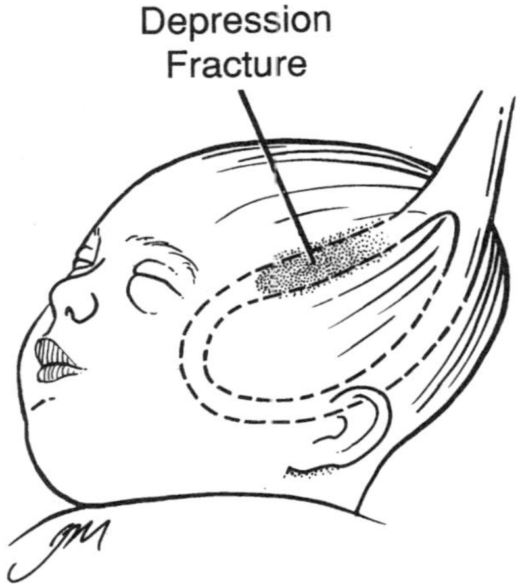

DEPRESSION FRACTURE

FIGURE 4

Depression fracture of the skull

Also caused by the use of forceps, is related to the development of epilepsy in early childhood. It is difficult to assess the resulting brain injury once the skull is fractured until the child is of nearly school age. (Figure 4).

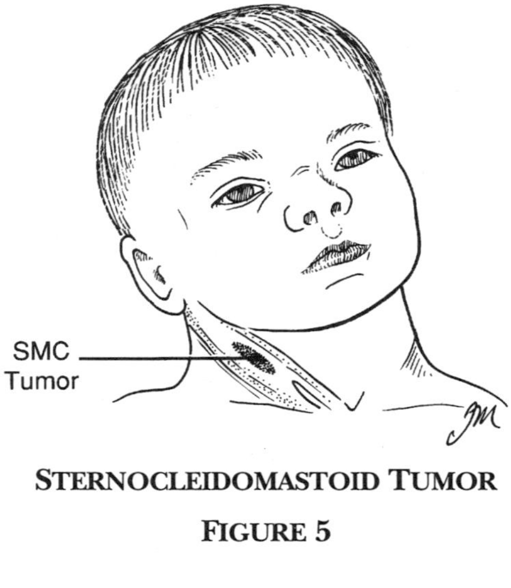

STERNOCLEIDOMASTOID TUMOR

FIGURE 5

Sternomastoid tumor

A painless lump in the SCM which appears after the first week of life due to trauma at birth. It is seen very frequently after a breech birth, and is almost always accompanied by torticollis (Figure 5). Chiropractic care of this condition can usually bring about a resolution to this problem in 2-3 weeks. Soft tissue work on the actual lump, which is no more than a muscular "knot", can aid in the resolution of the torticollis along with the adjustments.

Caput succedarum

"Normal" occurrence caused by the pressure of the cervix which interrupts the venous lymphatic drainage of the scalp. It is seen quite often in breech births where the largest cervical diameter is experienced last rather than first as with a vertex birth (Figure 6).

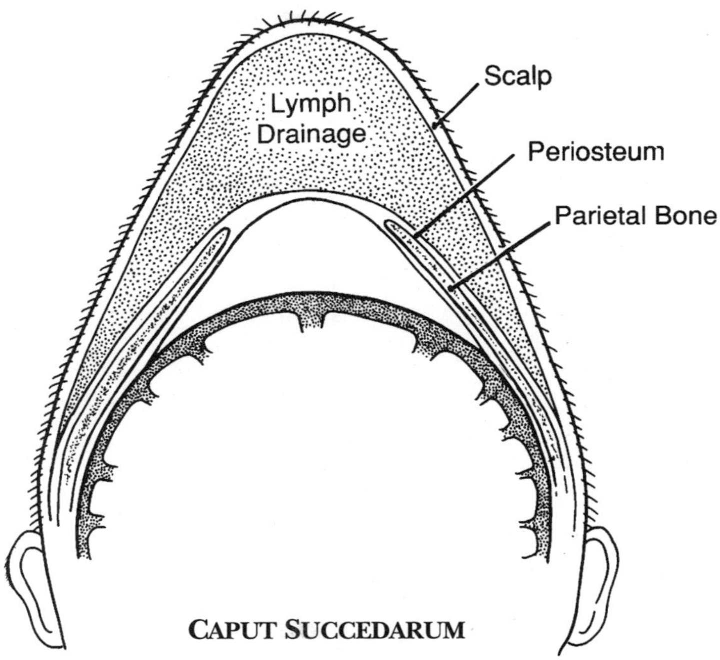

CAPUT SUCCEDARUM

FIGURE 6

Cephalohematoma

Pooling of blood between the periosteum and the skull bones is known as a cephalohematoma. It is normally limited to the area occupied by a cranial bone and does not cross the suture lines (Figure 7). The hemorrhage which is caused by trauma at birth is most often reabsorbed by the body in a few weeks. Should the hematoma cross a suture line, it is considered quite severe. ■

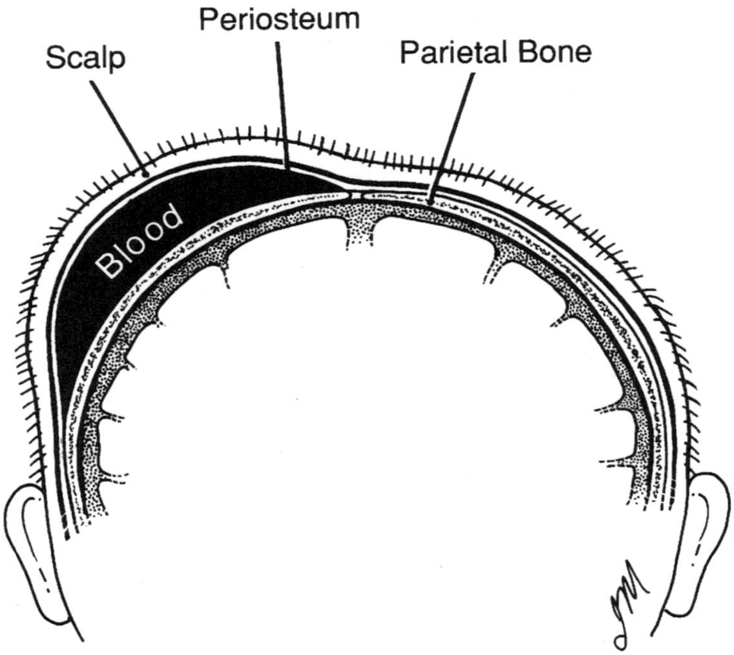

CEPHALOHEMATOMA

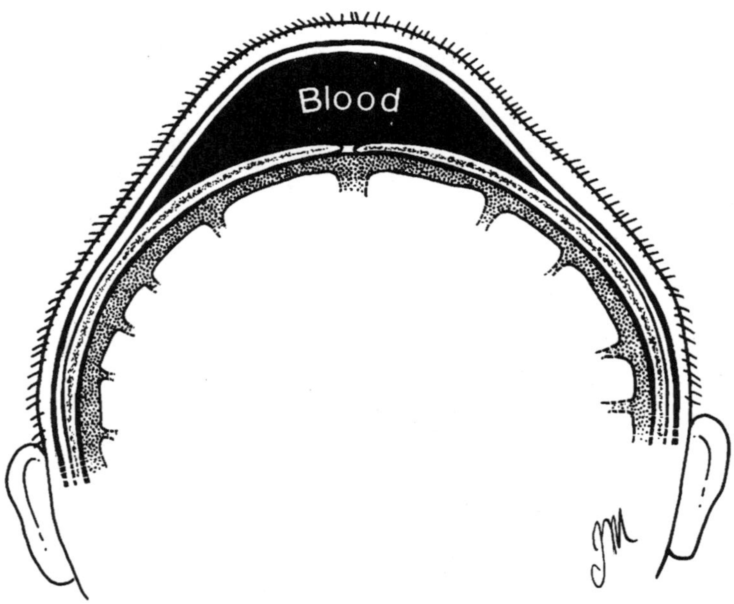

FIGURE 7

REFERENCES

Neonate

Anthony CL, Arnon R, Fitch CW: Pediatric Cardiology, Medical Outline Series. Medical Examination Publishing Co, Flushing N.Y., 1979

Barness LA: Manual of Pediatric Physical Diagnosis (4th ed.) Year Book Med, Chicago, 1972

Behrem RE (ed.): Neonatal-Perinatal Medicine (2nd ed), C.V. Mosby, St. Louis, 1977

Coleman SS: Congenital dysplasia and dislocation of the hip. C.V. Mosby, St. Louis, 1978

Cox D: The condyle subluxation in infants, Articles on pediatrics Vol II, International Review of Chiropractic, 1994

Kent C: An overview of pediatric radiology, Articles on Pediatrics Vol I, International Review of Chiropractic, 1994

Lovell WW, Winter RB: Pediatric Orthopaedics. J.B. Lippincott Co, Philadelphia, 1978

McMullen M: Assessing cervical subluxations in infants under six months of age. Articles on Pediatrics Vol I. International Review of Chiropractic, 1994

McMullen M: Handicapped children and chiropractic care (Part I & II). Articles on Pediatrics Vol 1. International Review of Chiropractic, 1994

Mellott S: Pediatric radiology, Articles on Pediatrics Vol II, International Review of Chiropractic, 1994

Roberts NK, Gelband H: Cardiac Arrhythmias in the neonate infant and child. Appleton-Century-Crofts, New York, 1977

Scarpelli EM, Auld PAM: Pulmonary Physiology of the Fetus Newborn and Child. Lea & Febiger, Philadelphia, 1975

Malpresentation

Amirikia H, Zarewych B, Evans TN: Cesarean section: A 15 year review of changing incidence, indications and risks. Am J Obstet Gynecol, 140:81, 1981

Bird GC: The use of the vacuum extractor. Clin Obstet Gynecol, 9:641, 1982

Collea JV, Rabin SC, Weghorst GR, et. al: The randomized management of term frank breech presentations: Vaginal delivery vs cesarean section. Am J Obstet Gynecol, 131:186, 1978

Cruikshank DP, White CA: Obstetric malpresentations: Twenty years experience. Am J Obst Gynecol, 116:1097, 1973

Dyson DC, Mellder PD, Armstrong MA: Management of prolonged pregnancy: Induction of labor versus antepartum fetal testing. Am J Obstet Gynecol, 156:928, 1987

Levine MG, Holroyde J, Woods JR, et al Birth trauma: Incidence and predisposing factors. Obstet Gynecol, 63:792, 1984

McMullen M: Assessing cervical subluxations in infants under six months of age. Articles on Pediatrics Vol I. International Review of Chiropractic, 1994

McMullen M: Handicapped children and chiropractic care (Part I, II). Articles on Pediatrics Vol1. International Review of Chiropractic, 1994

Ryden G: Vacuum extraction or forceps? (Editorial) Br Med J, 292:75 1986

Taffel SM, Placek PJ, Liss T: Trends in the United States caesarean section rate and reasons for the 1980-85 rise. Am J Pub Health, 77:955, 1987

Labor and Birth

Beazley JM: The active management of labor. Am J Obstet Gynecol, 122:161, 1975

Beck NC, Hall D: Natural childbirth: A review and analysis. Obstet Gynecol, 52:371, 1978

Capso AI: Force of labor. In Iffy L, Kaminetzky HA (eds.): Principles and practice of obstetrics and perinatology, John Wiley & Sons, New York, 1981

Carlson JM, Diehl JA, Sachtleben-Murray M, et.al.: Maternal positioning during parturition in normal labor. Clin Obstet Gynecol, 30:83, 1987

Danforth DN, Buckingham JC, Roddick JW: Connective tissue changes incident to cervical effacement. Am J Obstet Gynecol, 80:939, 1960

Freidman EA, Sachtleben MR, Bresky PA: Dysfunctional labor. XXI. Longterm effects of labor and delivery on offspring: A matched pair analysis. Am J Obstet Gynecol, 150:941, 1984

Ulmsten U, Ueland K (eds.): The forces of labor: Uterine contractions and the resistance of the cervix. Clin Obstet Gynecol, 26:1. 1983

Whittle MJ, Miller FC: The evaluation of uterine activity. Am J Obstet Gynecol, 136:38, 1980

Prenatal Testing

American College of Obstetricians and Gynecologists (ACOG): Technical Bulletin No.108. Antenatal diagnosis of genetic disorders. Washington, D.C. ACOG Meeting 1987

Cackle H, Wald NJ, Bankau G. et al: Biochemical screening for Downs syndrome. Lancet, 2:851, 1986

Campbell S: The assessment of fetal development by diagnostic ultrasound. Clin Perinatal, 1:2507, 1979

Fletcher JL: Update on pregnancy testing. Prin Care, 13:667, 1986

Glack L, Kulovich MV, Boner RC, et al: Diagnosis of respiratory distress syndrome by amniocentesis. Am J Obstet Gynecol, 109:440, 1971

Goldstein S: Vaginal endoscopy. Alan R Liss, New York, 1988

Rippey JH: Pregnancy tests: Evaluation and current status. CRC Crit Rev Clin Lab Sci, 19:353, 1984

Tabor A, Phillip J, Madsen M et al: Randomized controlled trials of genetic amniocentesis in 4606 low risk women. Lancet, 1:1287, 1986

Orthopedic/Neurological Conditions

Berg G, Hammar M, Moller-Nielsen J et al: Low back pain during pregnancy. Obstet and Gynecol, 72:71, 1988

Cohen BA, London RS, Goldstein PJ: Myastenia gravis and preeclampsia. Obstet and Gynecol, 48:35s, 1976

Davis FA: Impairment of repetitive impulse conduction in experimentally demyelinated and pressure injured nerves. J Neurol Neurosurg, Psychiatry, 39:443, 1972

Dalessio DJ: Classification and treatment of headache during pregnancy. Clinical Neuropharmocology, 9:121, 1986

Fallon JM: Orthopedic and neurological conditions of pregnancy, Multimedia Presentation, 1990

Fallon JM: The biomechanical and hormonal considerations of pregnancy as they relate to chiropractic care, Multimedia presentation 1989, 1993

Farfan HF: Mechanical Disorders of the Low Back, Lea & Febiger, Philadelphia, 1973

Gelb HGL: Clinical Management of Head, Neck and TMJ Pain and Dysfunction. Saunders, Philadelphia, 1977

Gilliatt RW: The cause of nerve damage in acute compression. Trans Am Neurol Assoc, 99:71, 1974

Haldemen S (ed): Modern Developments in the Principles and Practice of Chiropractic, Appleton-Century-Crofts, New York, 1980

Haldeman S: Interactions between the somatic and visceral nervous systems. ACA J Chiropractic, 5:57, 1971.

Hammar M, Larsson L, Tegler L:Calcium treatment of leg cramps in pregnancy. Acta Obstetrica et Gynecologia Scandinavica, 60:345, 1981

Homewood AE: The Neurodynamics of the Vertebral Subluxation. Valkyrie Press, St. Petersburg, 1979

Janse JH, Wells BF, et al: Chiropractic Principles and Technic, National College of Chiropractic, Chicago, 1947

Kopell HP: Help For Your Aching Back, Grosset & Dunlap, New York, 1969

LaBan MM, Perrin JCS, Latimer FR: Pregnancy and the herniated lumbar disc. Archives of Phy. Med and Rehabil. 64:320, 1983

Leach RA: The Chiropractic Theories, Williams & Wilkins, Baltimore, 1986

Lind GAM: Auto-Traction Treatment of Low Back Pain and Sciatica. Linkoping, Sweden, 1974

Lord JW Jr, Rosalie LM: Neurovascular Compression Syndromes of the Upper Extremity. Clin Symp, 23:2, 1971

Lowe TW, Weinreb J, Santos-Ramos R et al: Magnetic resonance imaging in human pregnancy. Obstet and Gynecol, 66:629, 1985

Lusted LB, Leats TE: Atlas of Roentgenographic Measurement. (2nd ed.) Chicago Yearbook, Chicago, 1967

MacGibbon B, Farfan HF: Are all lumbar spines the same- radiological survey. Spine, 4:258, 1979

Oswald I: Sudden body jerks on falling asleep. Brain, 82:92, 1959

Pacher AR, Steere AC: The triad of neurological manifestations of Lyme disease. Neurology, 35:47, 1986

Palmateer DC: Greater occipital-trigeminal syndrome. J Clin Chiropractic (arch ed.), Winter 1972

Poser S, Poser W: Multiple sclerosis and gestatation. Neurology 33:1422, 1983

Putti V: New conceptions in the pathogenesis of sciatic pain, Lancet, 2:53, 1927

Rainer GW, Mayer J, Sadler TR, Dirks D: Effects of graded compression on nerve conduction velocity. Arch Surg, 107:719, 1973

Reik L, Steere AC, Bartenhagen NH et. al.: Neurological abnormalities of Lyme disease without erythema chronicum migrans. Amer J of Medicine, 81:73, 1986

Schmorl G, Junghanns H: The Human Spine in Health and Disease (2nd ed.) Grune & Stratton, New York, 1971

Suh CH: Computer Aided Design Mechanisms. University of Colorado, Boulder, 1975

Wall PD, Waxman S, Basbaum AI: Ongoing activity in peripheral nerve: Injury discharge. Exp Neurol, 45:576, 1974

Wright DO, Patel MK: Focal migraine and pregnancy. British Med Journal, 293:1557, 1986

Anatomy & Physiology

Austin CR: Fertilization. Prentice-Hall, Englewood Cliffs, 1965

Austin CR: Sperm maturation in the male and female genital tracts. In Metz CB, Monray A (eds): Biology of Fertilization, Volume 2, Academic Press, New York, 1985

Braude P, Bolton V, Moore S: Human gene expression first occurs between the four- and eight-cell stages of the preimplantation development. Nature, 332:459, 1988

Braunstein GD, Rasor JL, Engvall E, et al: Interrelationships of human chorionic gonadatropin, human placental lactogen and pregnancy-specific glycoprotein throughout normal human gestation. Am J Obstet Gynecol, 138:1205 1980

Csapo AL, Pulkkinen MO: Indispensability of the human corpus luteum in the maintenance of early pregnancy luteectomy evidence. Obstet Gynecol Surv, 33:69 1978

Eastman NJ, Hellman LM: Williams Obstetrics, 13th ed. Appleton-Century-Crofts, New York, 1966

Fallon JM: Orthopedic and neurological conditions of pregnancy, Multimedia Presentation, 1990

Fallon JM: The biomechanical and hormonal considerations of pregnancy as they relate to chiropractic care, Multimedia presentation 1989, 1993

Gill TJ III, Immunity and Pregnancy. CRC Crit Rev Immunol, 5:201, 1985

Grant JCB: An Atlas of the Human Body. 7th ed. Williams and Wilkins, Baltimore, 1978

Hearn JP: The embryo-maternal dialogue during early pregnancy in primates. J Reprod Fertil, 76:809, 1986

Hunziker RD, Wegmann TG: Placental immunoregulation. CRC Crit Rev Immunol, 6:245 1987

Knobil E, Neill J (eds): The Physiology of Reproduction, Raven Press, New York, 1988

Lenton EA, Neal LM, Sulaiman R: Plasma concentrations of human chorionic gonadatropin from the time of implantation until the second week of pregnancy. Fertil Steril, 37:773 1982

Ludwig H, Metzer H, The Human Female Reproductive Tract. A Scanning Electron Microscope Atlas, Springer-Verlag, Heidelberg, 1976

McMullen M: Assessing cervical subluxations in infants under six months of age. Articles on Pediatrics Vol I. International Review of Chiropractic, 1994

Moore KL: The Developing Human, 4th ed. WB Saunders, Philadelphia, 1988

Pauerstein CJ, Hodgson BJ, Kramen MA: The anatomy and physiology of the oviduct. Obstet Gynecol Ann, 3:317 1974

Scott JR.,DiSaia PJ, Hammond CB.,Spellacy WN. Danforth's Obstetrics and Gynecology 6th ed. J.B. Lippincott Company, Philadelphia, 1990

Sholls HT, Orsini MW, Hitchins DJ: Estrogen synthesis and metabolism in the hamster blastocyst, uterus and liver near the time of implantation. J Steroid Biochemistry, 19:1153 1983

Ulfelder H: Mechanism of pelvic support in women. Am J of Obstet Gynecol, 72:856, 1956

Wynn RM(ed) Cellular Biology of the Uterus, Appleton-Century-Crofts, New York, 1967

Neuromuscular Skeletal System

Adour KK: The bell tolls for decompression? New England Journal of Medicine, 292:748, 1975

Aminoff MJ: Neurological disorders and pregnancy. Am J Obstet Gynecol, 132:325, 1978

Bell C: The Nervous System of the Human Body. Longman Rees, Orme, Brown, and Green, London, 1830

Berg G, Hammer M, Moller-Nielson J, et al: Low back pain during pregnancy. Obstetrics and Gynecology, 72:71

Berkwitz NJ and Lufkin NH: Toxic neuronitis of pregnancy: A clinicopathological report. Surgery, Gynecology and Obstetrics, 54:743, 1932

Benson RC, Inman VT: Brachialgia statica dysesthetica in pregnancy. Western Journal of Surgery, 64:115, 1956

Brown JT and McDougall A: Traumatic maternal birth palsy, Journal of Obstetrics and Gynecology of the British Empire, 64:431

Cole JT: Maternal obstetric paralysis, American Journal of Obstetrics and Gynecology, 52:386

Ecker AD and Woltman HW: Meralgia Parestetica: A report of one hundred and fifty cases, J Amer Med Assoc, 110: 1650, 1938

Eckman-Ordeberg G, Salgeback S, Ordeberg G: Carpal tunnel syndrome in pregnancy: A prospective study. Acta Obstet Gynecol Scand, 66:233, 1987

Fallon JM: Orthopedic and neurological conditions of pregnancy and chiropractic management of care, Articles on Pediatrics, Vol II, International Review of Chiropractic, 1994

Fallon JM: Orthopedic and neurological conditions of pregnancy, Multimedia Presentation, 1990, 1994

Fallon JM: The biomechanical and hormonal considerations of pregnancy as they relate to chiropractic care, Multimedia presentation 1989, 1993, 1994

Fisher AP, Hanna M: Transcutaneous nerve stimulation in meralgia parestetica of pregnancy, British J of Ob Gyn, 94:603, 1987

Font AT, Hankin RS: Pregnancy outcomes after now catastrophic maternal trauma during pregnancy. Obstet Gynecol, 35:912, 1970

Forster JB: Hydrocortisone and the carpal tunnel syndrome. Lancet, 1:456, 1960

Head HB, Welsh JS, Mussey E et al: Cyclic sciatica: Report of case with introduction of a new surgical sign. J Amer Med Assoc, 180:521, 1962

Hamlin E, Lehman RAW: Carpal Tunnel Syndrome, New Engl J Med, 276:849, 1967

Jones MW, Berry K: Chronic relapsing polyneuritis associated with pregnancy, Transactions of the Obstetrical Society of London, 9:12, 1981

Ironside R: Neuritis complicating pregnancy, Proceedings of the Royal Society of Medicine, 32:588, 1939

King G, Ride LT: The relation of vitamin B1 deficiency to pregnancy toxemias. J of Obstet Gynecol of the British Empire, 52:130, 1945

McMullen M: Assessing cervical subluxations in infants under six months of age. Articles on Pediatrics Vol I. International Review of Chiropractic, 1994

McMullen M: Handicapped children and chiropractic care (Part I & II). Articles on Pediatrics Vol 1. International Review of Chiropractic, 1994

O'Connell JEA: Lumbar disc protrusion in pregnancy. J of Neurology, Neurosurgery and Psychiatry, 23:138, 1960

Prineas J: Peripheral nerve changes in thiamine-deficient rats. Archives of Neurology, 23:541, 1970

Sands RX: Backache of pregnancy: a method of treatment. Obstet Gynecol, 12:670, 1958

Sommerville BW: A study of migraines in pregnancy. Neurology, 22:824, 1972

Strauss MB, McDonald WJ: Polyneuritis of pregnancy: A dietary deficiency disorder. J Amer Med Assoc, 100:1320, 1933

Robinson JR, Pou JW: Bell's Palsy: A predisposition of pregnant women. Archives of Otolaryngology, 95:125, 1972

Romberg MH: Diseases of the Nervous System Vol II, Sydenham Society, London, 1851

Urist MR: Obstetric fracture-dislocation of the pelvis: Report of a case with injury to the lumbosacral trunk and first sacral nerve roots. J Amer Med Assoc, 152:127, 1953

Systemic Changes During Pregnancy

Anderson LL: Regulation of relaxin secretion and it's role in pregnancy. Adv Exp Med Biol, 219:421, 1987

Baird JD: Some aspects of the metabolic and hormonal adaptation to pregnancy. Acta Endocrinol (suppl) (Copenh), 277:11, 1986

Brody SA, Ueland K (eds): Endocrine Disorders in Pregnancy, Appleton & Lange, Norwalk, 1989

Chesley LC, Sibai BM: Blood pressure in the midtrimester and future pre-eclampsia. Am J Obstet Gynecol, 157:1258,1987

Davison JM: Kidney function in pregnant women. Am J Kidney Disease 9:265, 1987

DeSwiet M: The Respiratory System. In Hytten FE, Chamberlain G(eds): Clinical Physiology in Obstetrics, 2nd ed. Blackwell, Oxford, 1991

Douvas SG, Meeks GR, Phillips JC, et al: Liver disease in pregnancy. Obstet Gynecol Surv, 38:531, 1983

Easterling TR, Schumucker BC, Benedetti TJ: The haemodynamic effects of orthostatic stress during pregnancy. Obstet Gynecol, 72:550, 1988

Fallon JM: Orthopedic and neurological conditions of pregnancy, Multimedia Presentation, 1990

Fallon JM: The biomechanical and hormonal considerations of pregnancy as they relate to chiropractic care, Multimedia presentation 1989, 1993

Gant NF, Whalley PJ, Everett RB, et al: Control of vascular reactivity in pregnancy. Am. J. Kidney Disease, 9:303, 1987

Grant JCB: An Atlas of the Human Body. 7th ed. Williams and Wilkins, Baltimore, 1978

Klein EA: Urologic problems in pregnancy: A review. Obstet Gynecol Surv, 39:605, 1984

Lind T: Metabolic changes in pregnancy relevant to diabetes mellitus. Postgrad Med J 55:353, 1979

Macfie AG, Magides AP, et al: Gastric emptying in pregnancy. Br J Anaesth, 67:54, 1991

Metcalfe J, McAnulty JH, Ueland K: Burwell and Metcalfe's Heart Disease in Pregnancy: Physiology and Management. Little, Brown, Boston, 1986

Milne JS, Howie AD, Pack AI: Dyspnoea during normal pregnancy. Br. J Obstet Gynaecol, 85:260, 1978

Pritchard JA, Scott DE: Iron stores of normal adults and their replenishment with oral iron therapy. J Amer Med Assoc, 190:897, 1964

Smout CFV, Jacoby F, Lillie EW: Gynecological and Obstetrical Anatomy. Williams and Wilkins, Baltimore, 1969

8 Congenital Malformations/ Genetic Defects/ Neonate Physiological Problems

There are many problems readily apparent at birth that will impact the neonate immediately. Some of those problems will be discussed here. The transition from the pregnancy to the care of the newborn happens rapidly, and the chiropractor should be aware of some of the problems that can present themselves from day one in the life of the neonate.

RESPIRATORY DISTRESS

Apnea

Some level of apnea is normal in the neonate for approximately 1-20 seconds. When it lasts longer than 20 seconds it becomes problematic and the neonate often dies. Statistics show that approximately 70% of apneic preemies will die, whereas only 15% of apneic full-term neonates will die.

Respiratory Distress Syndrome Type II

(Transient tachypenea of the newborn)

This is usually seen in full term newborns when there is a failure to completely evacuate the lung fluid at birth. It is seen soon after birth and lasts approximately 1-2 days. It is characterized by grunting, tachypenea, and retraction of the lungs. Chest films will reveal a generalized overexpansion of the lungs and a concomitant flattening of the diaphragm. Dense streaks are also visible in the hilar region denoting the remnants of fetal lung fluid.

Hyaline membrane disease

HMD will appear when the infant is born prior to the completion of the enzymatic pathways which produce surfactant. When the surfactant is lacking or is insufficient, the alveoli collapse and produce atelectasis. Due to the fact that diffuse atelectasis is present, blood that is traversing the lungs does not become fully oxygenated and the infant can become cyanotic and hypoxia. 20-25% of all premature infants experience this syndrome and of those 15-20% do not survive.

The fetal pathway for surfactant production begins to operate at approximately 22-24 weeks in utero, whereas the adult pathway of production does not begin until the 36th week in utero. A fetus that is born prior to the 36th week in utero will have difficulty with hyaline membrane disease.

S/S
- tachypenea
- retraction of chest wall
- dilatation of nasal alae/expiratory grunting
- Auscultation
  - diminished air exchange
  - harsh breath sounds
  - crepital rales

Hyperbilirubinemia/Jaundice

Excessive bilirubin may cause visible jaundice in the newborn. Old or damaged RBC's are removed from circulation by the reticuloendothelial cells. Newborns lack the intestinal bacteria for oxidizing bilirubin to some other products, therefore the way in which the bilirubin is broken down is two ways: (Figure 1)

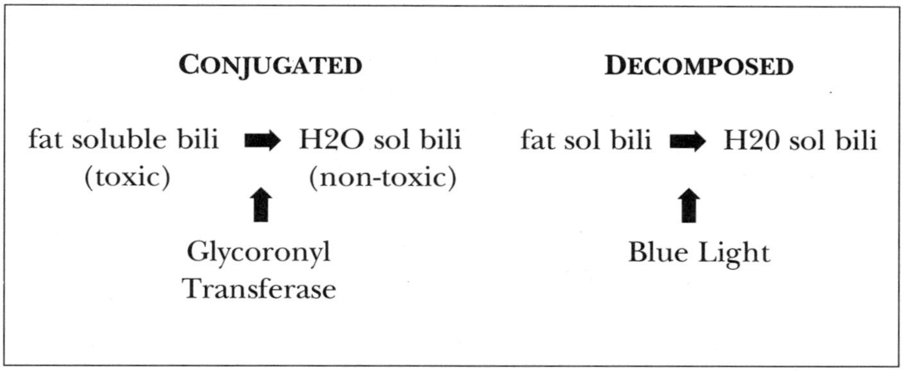

FIGURE 1

When there is fetal trauma, hemolytic disease or hematuria, there is the possibility of resulting jaundice. This is further encouraged when there is a decrease in gycoronyl transferase or biliary atresia. When liver function is impaired or inadequate it is termed obstructive jaundice. Non-obstructive jaundice can occur from immaturity, ABO or Rh incompatibility, excessive bruising or infection.

Treatment may consist of the following:

1) increase feedings which increase Gl motility and minimize the effects of the circulating bilirubin
2) phototherapy - photo-oxidizing bilirubin to the water soluble type
3) exchange transfusions

Congenital heart disease

Congenital abnormalities of the heart account for 10% of all neonatal deaths. 3-4% of all newborns possess a major heart anomaly, and by the age of five 7.5% of all children display some type of congenital heart defect.

Congenital heart disease appears in approximately 1 in 120 births. There are many factors which may contribute to the formation of congenital heart defects. Some of which are the following:

1) Genetic factors - inherited from the mother or father
2) Teratogenic Effects - drugs
   maternal illness
   infectious agents
   irradiation

3) Birth Process - maternal age difficult presentation difficult pregnancy/labor

S/S
- cyanosis
- murmur
- cardiomegaly
- arrhythmias
- cardiac situ
- delayed milestones
- congestive heart failure
- other congenital defects

Cleft Palate/Lip (Hare Lip)

This congenital malformation/full cleft palate (Figure 3) is often the result when the mother takes antiepileptic drugs when conception occurs. The lip is repaired at 4 months and the palate at about 1 year. These children have difficulty in sucking and may have to be spoon fed.

Occasionally the chiropractor will encounter a child with a bifid uvula (Figure 2). This is indicative of a cleft soft palate, where the hard palate is intact. Children who have a cleft soft palate will often experience bilateral otitis media far beyond the 18-24 month period. This is due most probably to the subluxative changes of the temporal and sphenoid bones of the child which result from the cleft in the soft palate.

Cleft Soft Palate (Bifid Uvula)

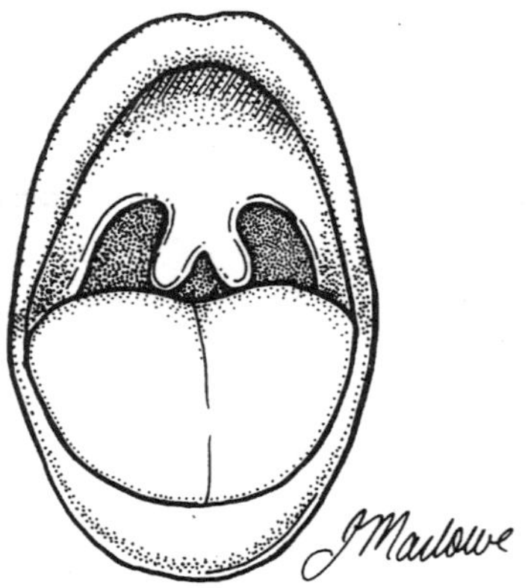

FIGURE 2

Full Cleft Palate

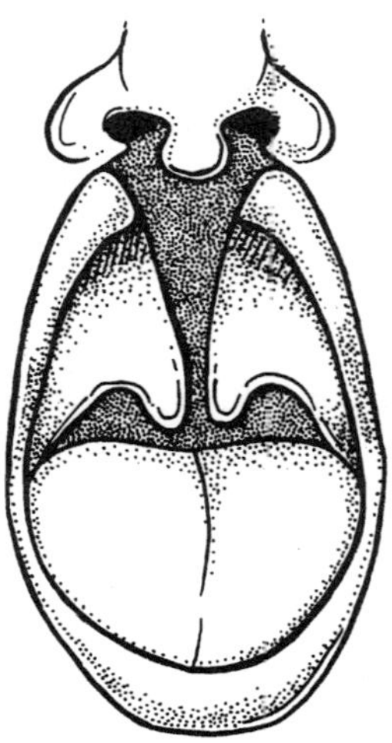

FIGURE 3

Esophageal atresia

When the newborn has difficulty swallowing and continues to keep spitting up with little or no milk being consumed, the possibility of an esophageal atresia must be considered. There is either a blind end to the esophagus or it can form a fistula with the trachea. When there is an unexplained hydramnios in utero the possibility of an esophageal atresia cannot be overlooked. It would signify that the fetus was unable to swallow amniotic fluid and therefore the amniotic fluid would have to be contained in the extra fetal space rather than within the fetus.

This is first suspected when the neonate begins to choke or aspirate when it is being fed.

- Blind pouch
- With tracheal fistula
- Memingocele/Meningomyelocele/Myelocele

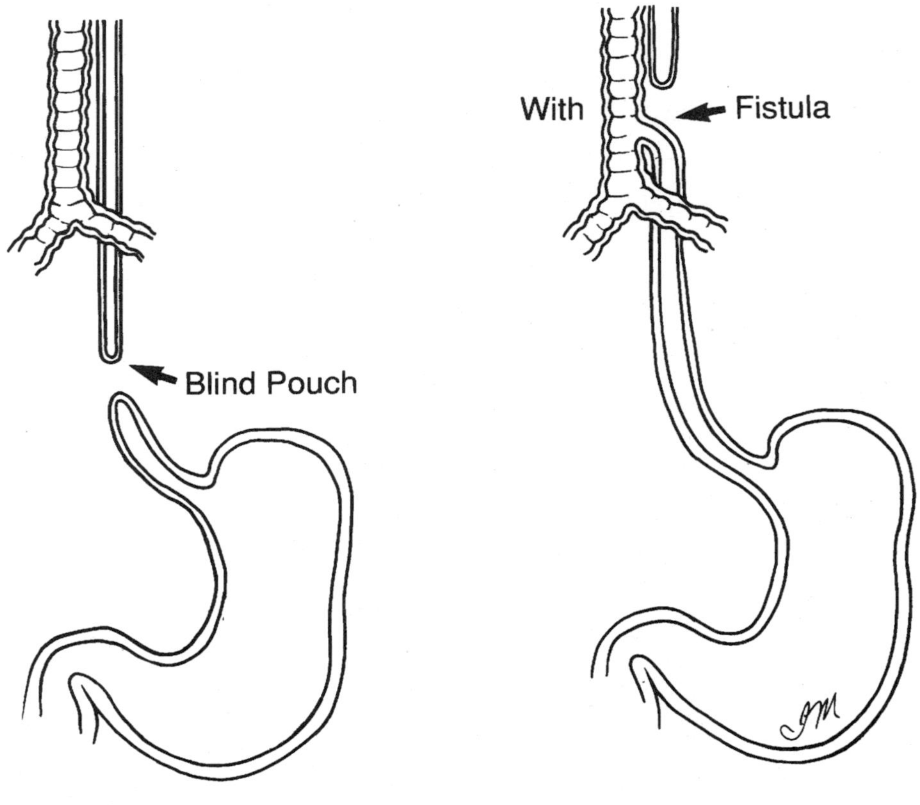

FIGURE 4

Meningocele

Herniation of the pia and arachnoid mater of the spinal cord. It is covered with skin and there is no cord displacement. Surgical closure is necessary but does not need to occur immediately. Most often the child will develop normally (Figure 5).

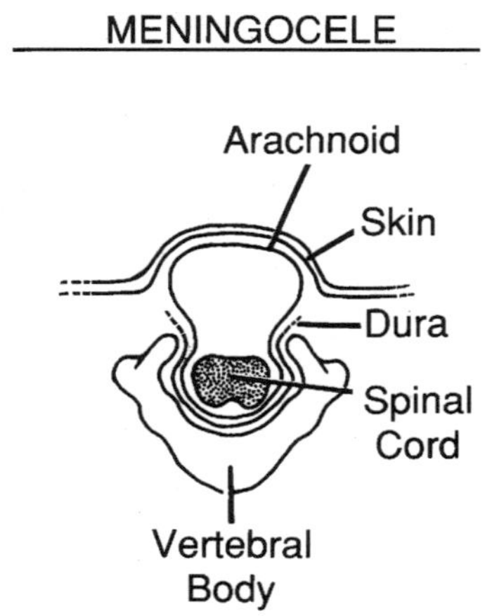

FIGURE 5

Meningomyelocele

The spinal cord is displaced as well as the surrounding sacs. The skin is incomplete and infection may set in therefore immediate closure is necessary. Paralysis of the bladder, bowel, legs and lower extremity may be present. Only one-third of these children survive without problems. The other two-thirds have significant problems with altered lifestyles (Figure 6).

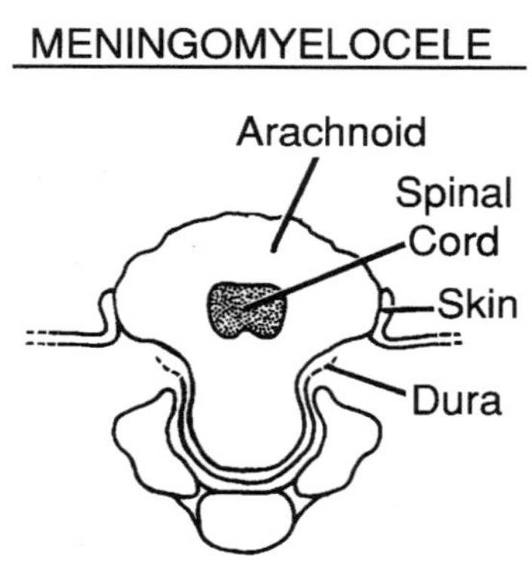

FIGURE 6

Myelocele

Here the entire spinal cord is exposed and it is not compatible with life. This type of malformation is often detected by ultrasonic examination in utero (Figure 7).

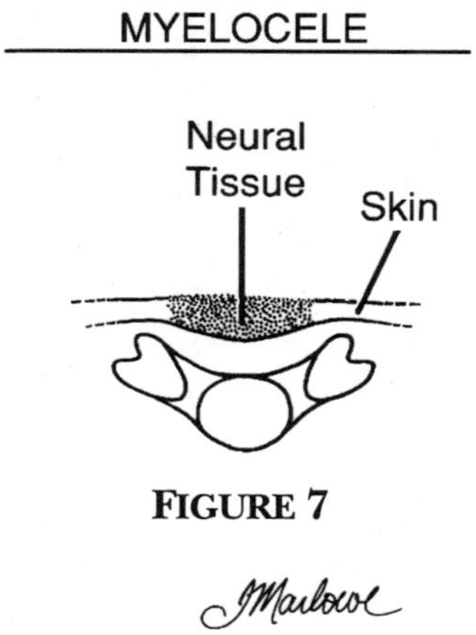

FIGURE 7

Accessory digits

Often times skin tags and or additional digits either fully or partially formed will present on the neonate. They can be easily removed and can signify a congenital or chromosomal defect as with achondroplasia where the newborn most often has a 6th digit on either the hands or the feet or both.

Talipes equinovarus

A common malformation usually caused by positioning in utero. Known more commonly as a club foot one or both feet are twisted inwards and the dorsum of the foot faces downwards. Often times it can be corrected with the proper adjustments but it is important for the doctor to be able to differentiate a true talipes from one of a positional stature. If one takes the foot and everts it and placing the sole downward, if there is a true talipes, the newborn will be unable to hold that position and the foot will revert to its original position. If on the other hand,

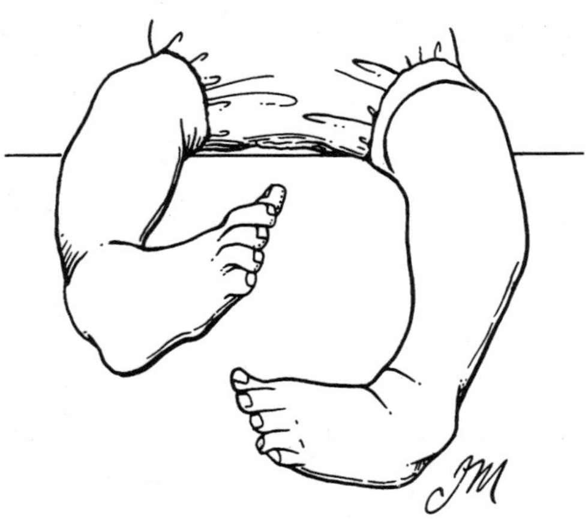

FIGURE 8

the child can maintain the position, there is less likelihood of it being a true talipes. Strapping techniques reinforcing the correct placement of the foot are often times effective in correcting the talipes.

Some of what the chiropractor will see which is diagnosed at birth as a talipes, is actually bony rotation of either the tibia or femur which responds very well to chiropractic care. Should surgery be needed, there are now new techniques being performed which when done prior to the 6th month can enable the child to crawl properly and not lose any developmental time.

Down's syndrome

The most common chromosomal abnormality in the neonate is Down's syndrome. Also known as Trisomy 21, it results from a nondysjunction of the chromosome 21 which corresponds to an extra chromosome on #21. Children born with this chromosomal abnormality show some similarities in phenotypic traits. Some characteristics are:

- upward slanting eyes
- Simian crease of the hand
- flattened occiput
- bridge nose
- lowered IQ
- hyptonia
- Buchfield's spots of the iris

Undescended testicle

Often times male newborns will present with one or more undescended testicle. Normally the testicle will descend within three months of birth. If it does not, then surgical referral may be necessary.

Hypospadias

In a male newborn occasionally one encounters a urethra that does not open at the tip of the penis but rather has its opening on the glands. (Figure 9) This does not require corrective surgery, but should the opening be in another place, surgical repair may be essential.

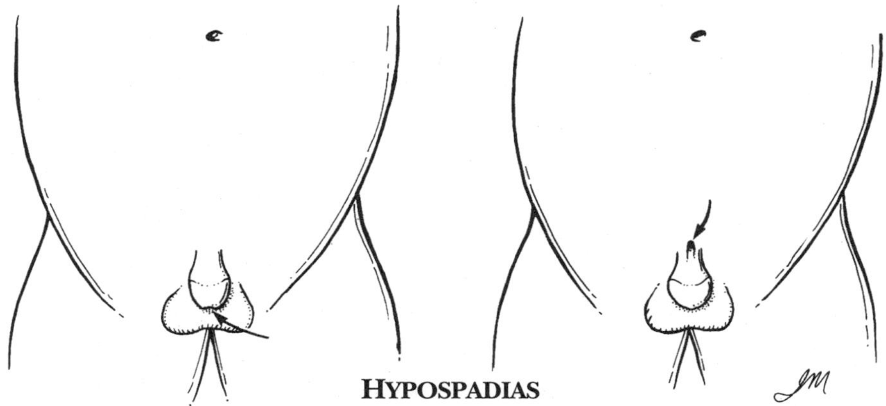

HYPOSPADIAS

FIGURE 9

Congenital dislocation of the hip

Encountered most frequently in the female newborn, it is thought to be because of the shape of the pelvis and the hormonal influences of the mother. Hip dislocation is detected by an orthopedic test known as Ortilani. The baby is placed supine on the examination table and the leg is flexed and the hip externally rotated until it touches the table. If there is a true hip dysplasia present, an audible click will be heard. This test should be performed at birth as well as 3-4 weeks later, and again at four months. It is important to perform this test prior to performing the reverse fencer reflex to determine subluxation in the newborn. ■

REFERENCES

Prenatal Testing

American College of Obstetricians and Gynecologists (ACOG): Technical Bulletin No.108. Antenatal diagnosis of genetic disorders. ACOG Meeting, Washington, D.C., 1987

Cackle H, Wald NJ, Bankau G. et. al.: Biochemical screening for Downs syndrome. Lancet, 2:851, 1986

Campbell S: The assessment of fetal development by diagnostic ultrasound. Clin Perinatal, 1:2,507, 1979

Fletcher JL: Update on pregnancy testing. Prin Care, 13:667, 1986

Glack L, Kulovich MV, Boner RC, et.al.: Diagnosis of respiratory distress syndrome by amniocentesis. Am J Obstet Gynecol, 109:440, 1971

Goldstein S: Vaginal endoscopy, Alan R Liss, New York, 1988

Rippey JH: Pregnancy tests: Evaluation and current status. CRC Crit Rev Clin Lab Sci, 19:353, 1984

Tabor A, Phillip J, Madsen M et al: Randomized controlled trials of genetic amniocentesis in 4606 low risk women. Lancet, 1:1287, 1986

Neonate

Anthony CL, Arnon R, Fitch CW: Pediatric Cardiology, Medical Outline Series. Medical Examination Publishing Co, Flushing N.Y., 1979

Barness LA: Manual of Pediatric Physical Diagnosis (4th ed.) Year Book Med, Chicago, 1972

Behrem RE (ed.): Neonatal-Perinatal Medicine (2nd ed), C.V. Mosby, St. Louis, 1977

Coleman SS: Congenital dysplasia and dislocation of the hip. C.V. Mosby, St. Louis, 1978

Cox D: The condyle subluxation in infants, Articles on Pediatrics Vol II, International Review of Chiropractic, 1994

Kent C: An overview of pediatric radiology, Articles on Pediatrics Vol I, International Review of Chiropractic, 1994

Lovell WW, Winter RB: Pediatric Orthopaedics. J.B. Lippincott Co, Philadelphia, 1978

McMullen M: Assessing cervical subluxations in infants under six months of age. Articles on Pediatrics Vol I . International Review of Chiropractic, 1994

McMullen M: Handicapped children and chiropractic care (Part I & II). Articles on Pediatrics Vol 1. International Review of Chiropractic. 1994

Mellott S: Pediatric radiology, Articles on Pediatrics Vol II, International Review of Chiropractic, 1994

Roberts NK, Gelband H: Cardiac Arrhythmias in the neonate infant and child. Appleton-Century-Crofts, New York, 1977

Scarpelli EM, Auld PAM: Pulmonary Physiology of the Fetus Newborn and Child. Lea & Febiger, Philadelphia, 1975

Congenital Abnormalities

Aase JM: Anticonvulsant drugs and congenital abnormalities. Amer J Disease of Children, 127:758, 1974

Anderson RC: Cardiac defects in children of mothers receiving anticonvulsant therapy during pregnancy. J of Pediatrics, 89:318, 1976

Bjeredal T: Epilepsy, Pregnancy and the Child. Raven Press, New York, 1982

Dansky LV, Andermann E, Rosenblatt D et. al.:Anticonvulsants, folate levels, and pregnancy outcome: A prospective study. Annals of Neurology, 21:176, 1987

McMullen M: Assessing cervical subluxations in infants under six months of age. Articles on Pediatrics Vol I . International Review of Chiropractic, 1994

McMullen M: Handicapped children and chiropractic care (Part I & II). Articles on Pediatrics Vol 1. International Review of Chiropractic, 1994

Nutrition

Begner L, Susser MW: Low birth weight and prenatal nutrition: An interpretive review. Pediatrics, 46:946, 1970

Fahey PJ, Boltri JM, Mark JS: Key issues on nutrition. From conception through infancy. Postgrad Med, 81:301, 1987

Hemminti E, Stanfield B: Routine administration of iron and vitamins during pregnancy: Review of controlled clinical trials. Br J Obstet Gynecol, 85:404, 1978

Jarnfelt-Samisoe A: Nausea and vomiting in pregnancy. A review. Obstet Gynecol Surv, 42: 422, 1987

National Research Council: Alternative Dietary Practices and Nutritional Abuses during Pregnancy. National Academy of Sciences, Washington D.C. 1982

Piconce TA, Allen LH, Olsen PN, Fern MF: Pregnancy outcome in North American women. Ill effects of direct cigarette smoking, stress, and weight gain on placentas and on neonatal physical and behavioral characteristics. Am J Clin Nutr, 36:1214, 1982

Bleeding During Pregnancy

Cotton DB, Read JA, Paul RH et al: The conservative aggressive management of placenta praevia. Am J Obstet Gynecol, 137:687, 1980

Post D: Vasa praevia. Am J Obstet Gynecol, 104:151,1979

Scott JR: Vaginal bleeding in the midtrimester of pregnancy. Am J Obstet Gynecol, 113:329, 1972

Effects of Therapeutic Drugs

Aase JM: Anticonvulsant drugs and congenital abnormalities. Amer J Disease of Children, 127:758, 1974

Anderson RC: Cardiac defects in children of mothers receiving anti-convulsant therapy during pregnancy. J of Pediatrics, 89:318, 1976

Callaghan N, Garrett A, Goggin T: Withdrawal of anticonvulsant drugs in patients free of seizures for two years. N Engl J Med, 318:942, 1988

Diggory PLC, Tomkinson JS: Nausea and vomiting in pregnancy: A trial of Meclizine dihydrochloride with and without pyridoxine Lancet, 2:370, 1962

Hartz SC, Heinonen OP, Shapiro S, et.al.: Antenatal exposure to meprobamate and chlordiazepoxide in relation to malformation, mental development, and childhood mortality. N Engl J Med, 292:726, 1975

Laegreid L, Olegard R, Wahlstrom J et.al.: Abnormalities in children exposed to benzodiazepines in utero. Lancet, 1:108, 1987

Mujtaba Q, Burrow GN: Treatment of Hyperthyroidism in pregnancy with propylthiouricil and Methimazole. Obstet Gynecol, 46:282, 1975

Nakane Y, Okuma T, Takahashi R, et.al.: Multi institutional study on the teratogenicity and fetal toxicity of antiepileptic drugs: A report of a collaborative study group in Japan. Epilepsia, 21:663, 1980

Rumeau-Rouquette C, Goujard J, Huel G: Possible teratogenic effect of phenothiazines in human beings. Teratology, 15:57, 1977

Safra MJ, Oakly GP:Association between cleft lip with or without cleft palate and prenatal exposure to diazepam. Lancet, 2:478, 1975

Neuromuscular Skeletal System

Adour KK: The bell tolls for decompression? New Eng J Med, 292:748, 1975

Aminoff MJ: Neurological disorders and pregnancy. Am J Obstet Gynecol, 132:325, 1978

Bell C: The Nervous System of the Human Body. Longman Rees, Orme, Brown, and Green, London, 1830

Berg G, Hammer M, Moller-Nielson J, et.al.: Low back pain during pregnancy. Obstetrics and Gynecology, 72:71

Berkwitz NJ and Lufkin NH: Toxic neuronitis of pregnancy: A clinicopathological report. Surgery, Gynecology and Obstetrics, 54:743, 1932

Benson RC, Inman VT: Brachialgia statica dysesthetica in pregnancy. Western Journal of Surgery, 64:115, 1956

Brown JT and McDougall A: Traumatic maternal birth palsy, J Obstet Gynecol of the British Empire, 64:431

Cole JT: Maternal obstetric paralysis, Am J Obstet and Gynecol, 52:386

Ecker AD and Woltman HW: Meralgia Parestetica: A report of one hundred and fifty cases, J Amer Med Assoc, 110:1650, 1938

Eckman-Ordeberg G, Salgeback S, Ordeberg G: Carpal Tunnel Syndrome in pregnancy. A prospective study. Acta Obstet Gynecol Scand, 66:233, 1987

Fallon JM: Orthopedic and neurological conditions of pregnancy and chiropractic management of care, Articles on Pediatrics Vol II, International review of Chiropractic, 1994

Fallon JM: Orthopedic and neurological conditions of pregnancy, Multimedia Presentation, 1990, 1994

Fallon JM: The biomechanical and hormonal considerations of pregnancy as they relate to chiropractic care, Multimedia presentation 1989, 1993, 1994

Fisher AP, Hanna M: Transcutaneous nerve stimulation in meralgia parestetica of pregnancy, British J of Ob Gyn, 94:603, 1987

Font AT, Hankin RS: Pregnancy outcomes after now catastrophic maternal trauma during pregnancy. Obstet Gynecol, 35:912, 1970

Forster JB: Hydrocortisone and the carpal tunnel syndrome, Lancet, 1:456, 1960

Head HB, Welsh JS, Mussey E et.al.: Cyclic sciatica: Report of case with introduction of a new surgical sign. J Am Med Assoc, 180:521, 1962

Hamlin E, Lehman RAW: Carpal Tunnel Syndrome, New Engl J Med, 276:849, 1967

Jones MW, Berry K: Chronic relapsing polyneuritis associated with pregnancy, Transactions of the Obstetrical Society of London, 9:12, 1981

Ironside R: Neuritis complicating pregnancy, Proceedings of the Royal Society of Medicine, 32:588, 1939

King G, Ride LT: The relation of vitamin B1 deficiency to pregnancy toxemias. J of Obstet Gynecol of British Empire, 52:130, 1945

McMullen M: Assessing cervical subluxations in infants under six months of age. Articles on Pediatrics Vol I. International Review of Chiropractic, 1994

McMullen M: Handicapped children and chiropractic care (Part I & II). Articles on Pediatrics Vol 1. International Review of Chiropractic, 1994

O'Connell JEA: Lumbar disc protrusion in pregnancy. J of Neurology, Neurosurgery and Psychiatry, 23:138, 1960

Prineas J: Peripheral nerve changes in thiamine-deficient rats. Archives of Neurology, 23:541, 1970

Sands RX: Backache of pregnancy: a method of treatment. Obstet Gynecol, 12:670, 1958

Sommerville BW: A study of migraines in pregnancy. Neurology, 22:824, 1972

Strauss MB, McDonald WJ: Polyneuritis of pregnancy: A dietary deficiency disorder. J Amer Med Assoc, 100:1320, 1933

Robinson JR, Pou JW: Bell's Palsy: A predisposition of pregnant women. Archives of Otolaryngology, 95:125, 1972

Romberg MH: Diseases of the Nervous System Vol II, Sydenham Society, London, 1851

Urist MR: Obstetric fracture-dislocation of the pelvis: Report of a case with injury to the lumbosacral trunk and first sacral nerve roots. J Amer Med Assoc, 152:127, 1953

9 Adjusting the Pregnant Woman

Adjusting the pregnant woman is one of the purest delights for the doctor of chiropractic. As mentioned elsewhere in the text, with the onset of any number of neuromuscular biomechanical problems that occur during pregnancy, chiropractic is extremely well-suited for the treatment of these conditions. In this chapter I will illustrate some of the techniques that can be used to adjust the pregnant woman. Each technique is well established in the chiropractic literature. My intent is not to exclude any technique but to simply propose some adjustments that the doctor of chiropractic can utilize in his or her practice. It is IMPORTANT however, that the doctor of chiropractic heed the clinical signs and symptoms that the pregnant woman presents with in the office prior to beginning any adjusting procedures. While clinical tests such as X-ray and MRI are contraindicated during pregnancy, one should always be alert to the possibility of a functional organic problem mimicking a subluxative change. Due to the fact that the hormonal levels alter the levels of pain and perception in the body of the pregnant woman, all conditions regardless of their etiology or prognosis, will be somewhat dampened in their presentation. In addition, internal problems such as appendicitis, fracture, tumor and infection will all have altered symptomotology.

Pelvis

Most of the problems that the pregnant woman will experience during the nine months of confinement occur in the surrounding areas of the pelvis. Muscles and ligaments which radiate in all directions from the pelvis are affected by the hormones of pregnancy. These effects on the pelvis have from a biomechanical point of view a tendency to become unstable. Subluxation at either or both of the SI (sacroiliac) joints as well as subluxation at the SP (symphysis pubis) joint can cause severe pain and discomfort during pregnancy.

Because of the extreme lordotic curve that is placed into the lumbar area due to the weight of the baby anteriorly, the pelvis will have a tendency to rock either forward AS (anterior-superior) and thus move with the lumbar vertebra, or in a more painful scenario, they will rock backwards either singly or together producing a PI (posterior-inferior) subluxation. Occasionally counter rotation is noted where one ilium rocks forward and the other rocks backward. This is often times seen in the young mother who is pregnant and also has a toddler. There is a tendency for the young mother to carry the toddler on one hip. This can create counter rotation. Two additional listing EX (external) and IN (internal) rotations are also seen.

Adjustments of the pelvis during pregnancy often times require ingenuity. There are chiropractic tables designed specifically with the pregnant woman in mind. A traditional Hi-lo, will allow the pregnant woman to lie completely prone due to the fact that the thoracic cushion falls away, thus allowing for the girth of the pregnant woman's abdomen. A pregnant woman, under normal circumstances, is unable to lie prone and she may find the position quite comfortable on the Hi-lo table.

The following are some of the adjustments done on the pelvis in pregnancy.

Adjusting the SP joint

The doctor stands on the side of the superior side of the subluxation.

The patient is placed supine. The doctor stands completely superior to the SP joint facing toward the feet. Either the drop mechanism on the Hi-lo table is raised or two pillows are placed under the buttocks of the patient to raise her up.

The fleshy pisiform of the doctor is placed on the superior portion of the SP joint, or the doctor can place his or her hand over the patient's which is placed directly on the SP joint. Those doctors or patients who feel uncomfortable with this adjustment can easily utilize this method.

If the SP joint on the right is subluxated the doctor will be standing on the right side of the patient with her right fleshy pisiform on the superior portion of the joint. Her left hand is then placed on top of the right for stabilization, and a slight thrust is given S-I (superior to inferior), and slight A-P anterior to posterior and in the direction of the left foot.

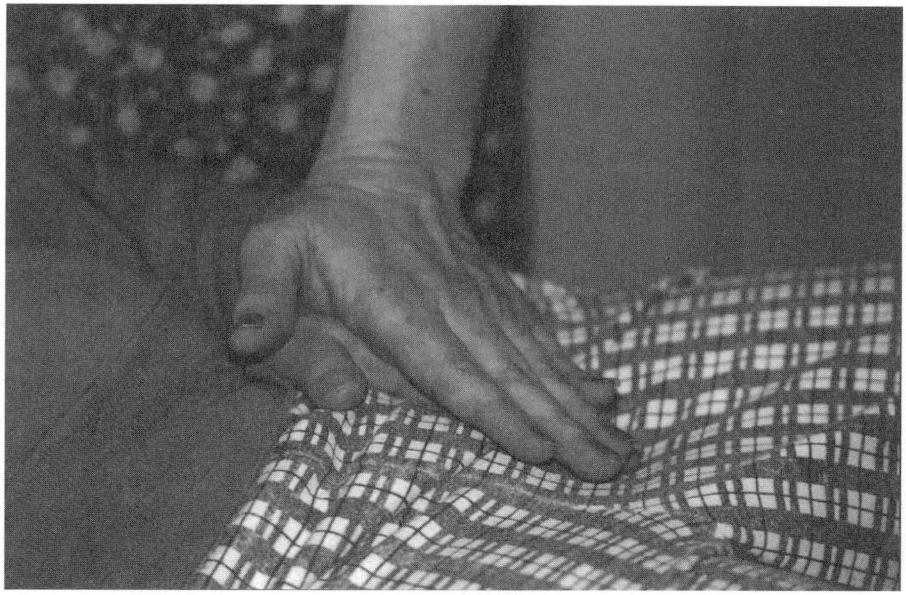

Adjusting the SI joint

PI (posterior inferior)

This adjustment can be made in either of two ways prone or side posture.

PRONE - with the patient prone and the Hi-lo adjusted for her abdominal girth, the doctor stands on the side of the subluxation.

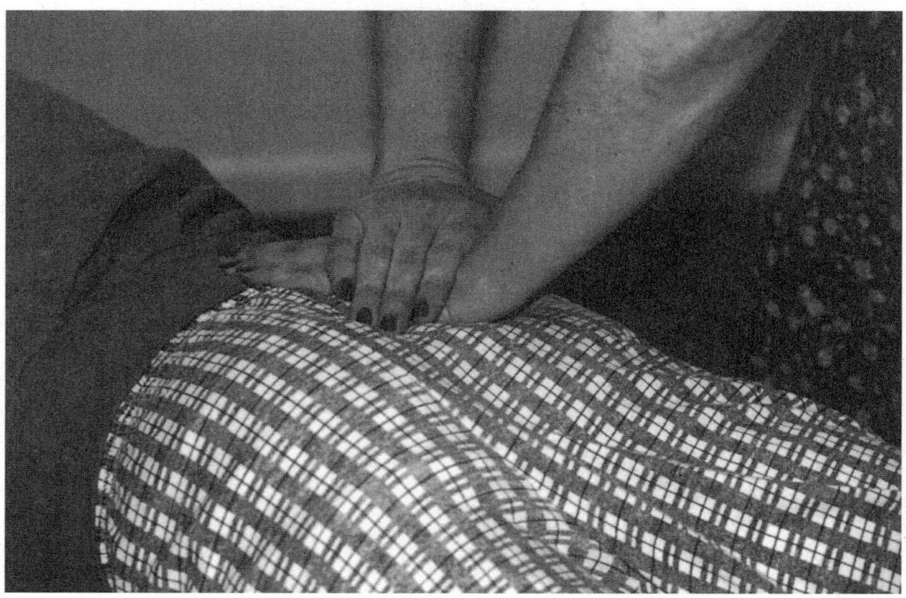

The inferior portion of the SI joint is contacted with the thenar emminence of the doctor hand. Assuming right sided PI, the doctor stands on the right side of the patient slightly inferior to the mid buttock area. With the fleshy part of the thenar eminence, on the right side, the doctor contacts the superior portion of the SI joint. The left hand is placed over the left SI joint for stabilization, and a thrust is given, I to S (inferior to superior) and P to A (posterior to inferior). It is important to note that the thrust is put only on one side of the body as it is a right sided PI. If both iliums are PI then the doctor must lean his or her body over the center of the patient and bilateral thrust is given.

AS (anterior superior)

This can also be adjusted either prone or side posture.

PRONE– In the prone position, the doctor stands superior to the mid-buttock region. Assuming a right sided AS the doctor stands on the right side of the patient, and contacts the posterior aspect of the ishial tuberosity with the thumb web of the left hand. The right hand is placed around the wrist for stabilization. The Hi-lo table's pelvic piece is cocked with the proper tension, and the thrust is given S to I and P to A in a rocking motion.

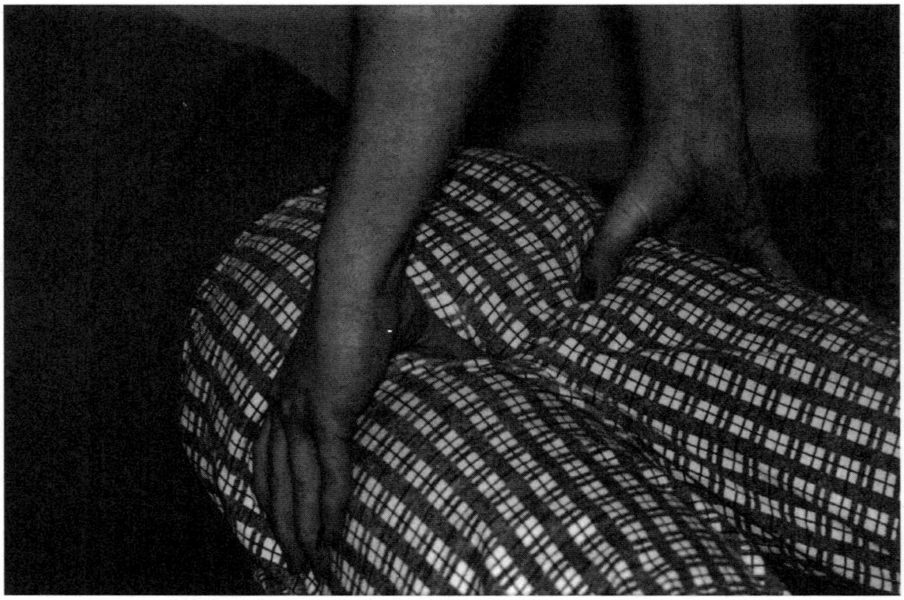

Side posture

Side posture moves can be easily performed on the pregnant woman. It is important to remember that the connective tissue is more supple and the point of tension will most likely be different in the pregnant woman. It should be noted that proper technique is important to maintain so as not to increase the amount of stretch applied to the motor units. Should the torque and stretch on the supporting structures become too great, the doctor risks increasing the possibility of inducing disk herniation. If the side posture moves are done correctly, there is no risk of this problem occurring.

Ex & In

These listings can be adjusted in accordance with whatever technique the doctor generally uses.

Lumbar spine

The lumbar spine can be adjusted either prone or side posture. In fact many doctors prefer to use a knee chest table during pregnancy to adjust the lumbar and thoracic spine. Assuming proper patient position, this technique can be utilized throughout the pregnancy. Indeed many pregnant women find the knee chest position extremely comfortable during pregnancy and often times give birth in that position.

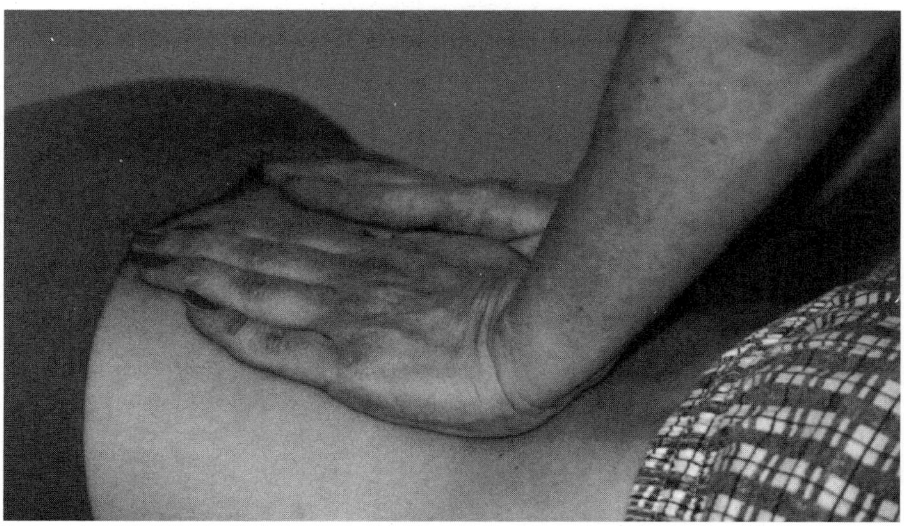

Thoracic spine

As discussed earlier, the thoracic spine is probably the first area of the spine to be affected during pregnancy. During the first three months of pregnancy, the thoracic spine undergoes tremendous attitudinal changes which can place the transverse process/rib head articulation in the new juxtaposition. This may cause severe pain in the thoracic region. In addition, rotational movements of the thoracic spine may be seen along with other subluxation types.

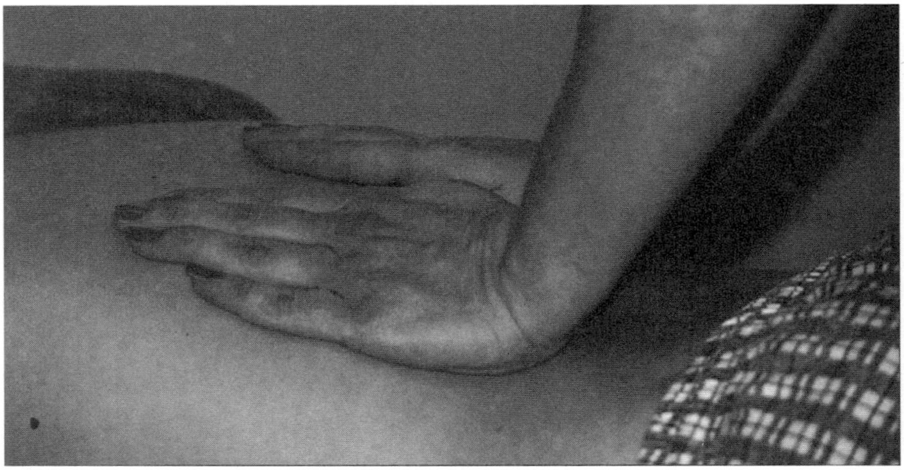

Cervical spine

Subluxations of the cervical spine can be involved in certain conditions seen during pregnancy such as brachial neuralgia. Often, the cervical spine has less subluxative problems than other places in the spine due to the fact that there are more stabilizing factors within it. Since it is farthest removed from the majority of the weight gain experienced during pregnancy, the cervical spine maintains its integrity better than the thoracic or lumbo-pelvic region. One problem that does exist however, is that due to the hormonal changes that occur, chiropractors will find themselves using more rotation, and lateral bending and stretching, to find the point of tension before delivering an osseous adjustment. This should be guarded against and should be considered prior to adjusting the pregnant woman.

Cranial bones

While some in our profession do not include the cranium as part of the spine, I think that it is important for us to consider it here. One of the major areas of subluxation-induced neurological problems encountered during pregnancy is Bell's Palsy. The cranium most certainly needs to be included as a location for subluxation. Subluxation may occur in the cranium as a result of the hormonal changes that occur during pregnancy, or as a result of trauma during the labor and delivery of the child. It is important to examine the clinical aspects of Bell's palsy to see when it occurred and is it likely to be a result of cranial bone involvement.

Extremity adjusting

As stated earlier, there are many extremity based conditions such as carpal tunnel syndrome that can occur in the pregnant woman as a result of hormonal changes which can induce subluxation. Each case needs to be examined on an individual basis. One must understand the movement of the extremity joints in the non-pregnant state in order to determine if there is true subluxation at the extremity during pregnancy. The joints are too numerous to discuss on an individual basis, as so many of the joints can potentially become involved. Extremity joints that are likely to experience subluxative changes during pregnancy are:

Wrist	most common site
Elbow	
Calcaneus/talus	
Ankle	
Shoulder	
Knee	least common site

REFERENCES

Adjusting the Pregnant Woman

DeBoer KF, Harmon RO, Savoie, Tuttle CD: Inter and intra-examiner reliability of leg length differential measurement: a preliminary study. J Manip Physiolog Ther, 6:61, 1983

Fallon JM: Chiropractic and Pregnancy, Articles on Pediatrics Vol I, International Review of Chiropractic, 1994

Fallon JM: Orthopedic and neurological conditions of pregnancy, Multimedia Presentation, 1990

Fallon JM: Orthopedic and neurological conditions of pregnancy and chiropractic management of care, Articles on Pediatrics Vol II, International Review of Chiropractic, 1994

Fallon JM: The Biomechanical and hormonal considerations of pregnancy as they relate to chiropractic care, Multimedia presentation 1989, 1993

Finneson BE (ed): Low Back Pain. Lippincott, Philadelphia, 1980

Grostic J: Some observations on computer-aided x-ray analysis. International Review of Chiropractic, 33:38,1979

Haldeman S: Spinal Manipulative Therapy. Clin Orthop, 179:62, 1983

Hamlin E, Lehman RAW: Carpal Tunnel Syndrome, New Engl J Med, 276:849, 1967

Ironside R: Neuritis complicating pregnancy, Proceedings of the Royal Society of Medicine, 32:588, 1939

Palmer DD: The Science, Art and Philosophy of Chiropractic, Portland Printing House, Portland, 1910

Palmer MH: Chiropractic Anatomy Vol IX, Palmer College of Chiropractic, Davenport, 1929

Ulfelder H: Mechanism of pelvic support in women. Am J of Obstet Gynecol, 72:856, 1956

Post Partum Depression

Fondeur M, Vixsen C, Triebel WA et.al.: Postpartum mental illness: A controlled study. Archives of Neurology and Psychiatry, 77:503, 1957

LLoyd JH Puerpural insanity and the insanity of pregnancy and lactation. A System of Obstetrics. Vol 2. Lea Brothers, Philadelphia, 1889

Robin AA: The psychological changes of normal parturition. Psychiatric Quarterly, 36:129, 1962

Zilborg G: Depressive reactions related to parenthood. American J of Psychiatry, 10:927, 1931

Orthopedic/Neurological Conditions

Berg G, Hammar M, Moller-Nielsen J et al: Low back pain during pregnancy. Obstet and gynecol, 72:71, 1988

Cohen BA, London RS, Goldstein PJ: Myastenia gravis and preeclampsia. Obstet and Gynecol, 48:35s, 1976

Davis FA: Impairment of repetitive impulse conduction in experimentally demyelinated and pressure injured nerves. J Neurol Neurosurg Psychiatry, 39:443, 1972

Dalessio DJ: Classification and treatment of headache during pregnancy. Clinical Neuropharmocology, 9:121, 1986

Fallon JM: Orthopedic and neurological conditions of pregnancy, Multimedia Presentation, 1990

Fallon JM: The biomechanical and hormonal considerations of pregnancy as they relate to chiropractic care, Multimedia presentation 1989, 1993

Farfan HF: Mechanical Disorders of the Low Back, Lea & Febiger, Philadelphia, 1973

Gelb HGL: Clinical Management of Head, Neck and TMJ Pain and Dysfunction. Saunders, Philadelphia, 1977

Gilliatt RW: The cause of nerve damage in acute compression. Trans Am Neurol Assoc, 99:71, 1974

Haldemen S (ed): Modern Developments in the Principles and Practice of Chiropractic, Appleton-Century-Crofts, New York, 1980

Haldeman S: Interactions between the somatic and visceral nervous systems. ACA J Chiropractic, 5:57, 1971.

Hammar M, Larsson L, Tegler L: Calcium treatment of leg cramps in pregnancy. Acta Obstetrica et Gynecologia Scandinavica, 60:345, 1981

Homewood AE: The Neurodynamics of the Vertebral Subluxation. Valkyrie Press, St. Petersburg, 1979

Janse JH, Wells BF, et al: Chiropractic Principles and Technic, National College of Chiropractic, Chicago, 1947

Kopell HP: Help For Your Aching Back, Grosset & Dunlap, New York, 1969

LaBan MM, Perrin JCS, Latimer FR: Pregnancy and the herniated lumbar disc. Archives of Phy. Med and Rehabil, 64:320, 1983

Leach RA: The Chiropractic Theories, Williams & Wilkins, Baltimore, 1986

Lind GAM: Auto-Traction Treatment of Low Back Pain and Sciatica. Linkoping, Sweden, 1974

Lord JW Jr, Rosalie LM: Neurovascular Compression Syndromes of the Upper Extremity. Clin Symp, 23:2, 1971

Lowe TW, Weinreb J, Santos-Ramos R et.al.: Magnetic resonance imaging in human pregnancy. Obstet and Gynecol, 66:629, 1985

Lusted LB, Leats TE: Atlas of Roentgenographic Measurement. (2nd ed.) Chicago Yearbook, Chicago, 1967

MacGibbon B, Farfan HF: Are all lumbar spines the same- radiological survey. Spine, 4:258, 1979

Oswald I: Sudden body jerks on falling asleep. Brain, 82:92, 1959

Pacher AR, Steere AC: The triad of neurological manifestations of Lyme disease. Neurology, 35:47, 1986

Palmateer DC: Greater occipital-trigeminal syndrome. J Clin Chiropractic (arch ed.), Winter, 1972

Poser S, Poser W: Multiple sclerosis and gestatation. Neurology, 33:1422, 1983

Putti V: New conceptions in the pathogenesis of sciatic pain, Lancet, 2:53, 1927

Rainer GW, Mayer J, Sadler TR, Dirks D: Effects of graded compression on nerve conduction velocity. Arch Surg, 107:719, 1973

Reik L, Steere AC, Bartenhagen NH et. al.: Neurological abnormalities of Lyme disease without erythema chronicum migrans. Amer J of Medicine, 81:73, 1986

Schmorl G, Junghanns H: The Human Spine in Health and Disease (2nd ed.) Grune & Stratton, New York, 1971

Suh CH: Computer Aided Design Mechanisms. University of Colorado, Boulder, 1975

Wall PD, Waxman S, Basbaum AI: Ongoing activity in peripheral nerve: Injury discharge. Exp Neurol, 45:576, 1974

Wright DO, Patel MK: Focal migraine and pregnancy. Br Med J, 293:1557, 1986

Malpresentation

Amirikia H, Zarewych B, Evans TN: Cesarean section: A 15 year review of changing incidence, indications and risks. Am J Obstet Gynecol, 140:81, 1981

Bird GC: The use of the vacuum extractor. Clin Obstet Gynecol, 9:641, 1982

Collea JV, Rabin SC, Weghorst GR, et.al: The randomized management of term frank breech presentations: Vaginal delivery vs cesarean section. Am J Obstet Gynecol, 131:186, 1978

Cruikshank DP, White CA: Obstetric malpresentations: Twenty years experience. Am J Obst Gynecol, 116:1097, 1973

Dyson DC, Mellder PD, Armstrong MA: Management of prolonged pregnancy: Induction of labor versus antepartum fetal testing. Am J Obstet Gynecol, 156:928, 1987

Levine MG, Holroyde J, Woods JR, et. al. Birth trauma: Incidence and predisposing factors. Obstet Gynecol, 63:792, 1984

McMullen M: Assessing cervical subluxations in infants under six months of age. Articles on Pediatrics Vol I. International Review of Chiropractic, 1994

McMullen M: Handicapped children and chiropractic care (Part I & II). Articles on Pediatrics Vol 1. International Review of Chiropractic, 1994

Ryden G: Vacuum extraction or forceps? (Editorial) Br Med J, 292:75 1986

Taffel SM, Placek PJ, Liss T: Trends in the United States caesarean section rate and reasons for the 1980-85 rise. Am J Pub Health, 77:955, 1987

Systemic Changes During Pregnancy

Anderson LL: Regulation of relaxin secretion and its role in pregnancy. Adv Exp Med Biol, 219:421, 1987

Baird JD: Some Aspects of the metabolic and hormonal adaptation to pregnancy. Acta Endocrinol (suppl) (Copenh), 277:11, 1986

Brody SA, Ueland K (eds): Endocrine Disorders in Pregnancy, Appleton & Lange, Norwalk, 1989

Chesley LC, Sibai BM: Blood pressure in the midtrimester and future pre-eclampsia. Am J Obstet Gynecol, 157:1258, 1987

Davison JM: Kidney function in pregnant women. Am J Kidney Dis, 9:265, 1987

DeSwiet M: The respiratory system. In Hytten FE, Chanberlain G (eds): Clinical Physiology in Obstetrics, 2nd ed. Oxford, Blackwell 1991

Douvas SG, Meeks GR, Phillips JC, et.al.: Liver disease in pregnancy. Obstet Gynecol Surv, 38:531, 1983

Easterling TR, Schumucker BC, Benedetti TJ: The haemodynamic effects of orthostatic stress during pregnancy. Obstet Gynecol, 72:550, 1988

Fallon JM: Orthopedic and neurological conditions of pregnancy, Multimedia Presentation, 1990

Fallon JM: The Biomechanical and hormonal considerations of pregnancy as they relate to chiropractic care, Multimedia presentation 1989, 1993

Gant NF, Whalley PJ, Everett RB, et.al.: Control of vascular reactivity in pregnancy. Am. J. Kidney Disease, 9:303, 1987

Grant JCB: An Atlas of the Human Body. 7th ed. Williams and Wilkins, Baltimore, 1978

Klein EA: Urologic problems in pregnancy: A review. Obstet Gyecol Surv, 39:605, 1984

Lind T: Metabolic changes in pregnancy relevant to diabetes mellitus. Postgrad Med J, 55:353, 1979

Macfie AG, Magides AP, et. al.: Gastric emptying in pregnancy. Br J Anaesth, 67:54, 1991

Metcalfe J, McAnulty JH, Ueland K: Burwell and Metcalfe's Heart Disease in Pregnancy: Physiology and Management. Little, Brown, Boston, 1986

Milne JS, Howie AD, Pack AI: Dyspnoea during normal pregnancy. Br J Obstet Gynaecol, 85:260, 1978

Pritchard JA, Scott DE: Iron stores of normal adults and their replenishment with oral iron therapy. JAMA, 190:897, 1964

Smout CFV, Jacoby F, Lillie EW: Gynecological and Obstetrical Anatomy. Williams and Wilkins, Baltimore, 1969

10 Case Reports

A 12-week pregnant woman with mid back pain

A 12-week pregnant woman presents in the office with pain in the mid back that she describes as unrelenting. Previously she had been to the obstetrician and it was explained to her that transient pain during pregnancy is not uncommon, and that she could apply heat to the back and if that didn't work she could try an ice pack.

History

Meg is a 32-year-old 12 week pregnant woman who presented with mid back pain. This is her third pregnancy and she describes that while she had some pain in her hips during her first two pregnancies and what was described to her as sciatica during her second pregnancy, she never had pain of this magnitude and that it scared her. Her first two pregnancies resulted in two live births the first in 1985, a boy, and the second in 1988 which was a girl. Each child ages 9 and 6 are reported to be in excellent health. Her first pregnancy went to 42 weeks and she had a hospital vaginal birth with a labor duration of 19 hours. Her second pregnancy went to 40 weeks, and she had a hospital vaginal birth with a labor of 13 hours. Neither pregnancy was complicated, and she denied using any type of anesthesia or drugs during either birth.

Meg reports her overall health to be excellent. She denies any physical or mental disabilities and denies any drug, alcohol or smoking. Her parents are both living with her mother age 56 and in reported good health, and her father age 57 also reported to be in good health with some slight hypertension which is controlled with diet.

Her mid back pain began eight days ago and continually became worse over time. It began as an ache on day one and gradually turned into a dull throbbing pain on the right side. The pain becomes worse when she takes a deep breath and does not seem to bother her on expiration. None of the strategies given to her by the obstetrician seem to work. The heat apparently makes it worse and the cold numbs it for approximately an hour and the pain comes right back. Some of the worst pain comes when she lies down at night.

Examination

Meg appears as a well developed, well nourished 32-year-old multipara who is 12 weeks pregnant. Physical exam including ENT, cardiovascular, fundascopic, and GI were well within normal limits. She exhibited some slight tenderness upon left upper quadrant palpation, which was thought to relate to her slight nausea, which she forgot to mention as part of the case history. Orthopedic and neurological examination too were within normal limits including laseque, Braggards, Hibb, cervical depression, shoulder depressor, and Soto Hall. Reflexes including biceps, triceps, brachioradialis, and jaw were +1 (0-+2). Meg was able to do moves through a full range of motion with a notable exception being that there was some slight tenderness upon right lateral bending at the waist.

Chiropractic Examination

Static and motion palpation of the cervical and lumbar spine was within normal limits and elicited no pain. Motion palpation of the thoracic spine similar to the range of motion exercise that Meg was put through elicited some slight pain upon movement on the right side. Anterior to posterior movement of the thoracic spine T4-T10 was most painful and most restrictive. Static palpation of the mid thoracic spine T3-T8 elicited pain over the thoraco-costal junction on the right side.

Treatment

Meg was placed on the Hi-lo prone and her subluxations at T4 and T8 were adjusted (diversified PL) by standing on the right side of the patient and with the doctor's right thumb taking a tissue pull from the spinous process of T4 out to the transverse process of T4. The doctor then places her or her left fleshy pisiform on the transverse process of T4 with the fingers pointing up the spine toward the head. The right fleshy pisiform is then placed on the left transverse process of T4 for stabilization. A posterior to anterior, inferior to superior thrust is then applied. T8 (PL) was similarly adjusted with correction made for the differing part of the spine.

Meg was seen again in one week and again a week later. She was administered the following adjustments during her subsequent two visits:

WEEK 2: T6 PL C2 PRS

WEEK 3: C2 PRS

Discussion

It is clear that Meg was suffering from intercostal neuralgia due to the changing attitude of the rib cage experienced early in pregnancy. Meg was classically affected due to the fact that this was her third pregnancy. Because there is a need for increased tidal volume and inspiratory and expiratory volume during pregnancy, one of the major accommodations that the body makes is to change the attitude of the ribcage, by flattening the diaphragm, and blunting the costophrenic angles. These changes allow for an increase in the functioning of the respiratory system. This process is facilitated and made possible by the large increase in estrogen and progesterone in the pregnant woman. The presence of increased quantities of these hormones produces a laxity of the ligaments, and a subsequent alteration of the supporting structures of the body.

One very important consideration here is to examine the differential diagnosis of this problem. While it is easy to see that in Meg's case this was purely a subluxative problem, there are problems which could mimic this type of pain. The presence of the increases in estrogen and progesterone in addition to producing alteration in structures also produce a type of anesthesia for the pregnant woman and her pain perception becomes altered. Any type of pain present, must be examined with an eye towards the fact that her perception of pain is altered and may be more serious than appears on the surface. In this case it would be important to rule out any type of lung problem for Meg such as pneumonia or even embolism.

Conclusion

Meg's condition completely cleared after two adjustments. While her third visit revealed no further subluxations present in her thoracic spine, Meg continued her visits on a monthly basis, until her third trimester when she was seen weekly. During her 41st week and 42nd week of gestation she was seen twice a week. She delivered a 8 lb. 2 oz. girl after an eight hour labor. Meg continues as a patient in the office as do now her three children.

A 38-week pregnant woman with sciatica

Jane presented in the office limping on her right leg holding her lower back as she walked into the office. Her midwife diagnosed sciatica and sent her in to be adjusted after first calling the office and describing the condition.

History

Jane is a 25-year-old 38 week primigravida who presented in the office complaining of previously diagnosed sciatic neuralgia. Her midwife's diagnosis appeared to be consistent with her presentation of a right sided limp and slight antalgia to the left and pain radiating down her right leg. Jane reported that this is her second pregnancy in the last three years with the first pregnancy resulting in miscarriage after eight weeks. Jane reported that this pregnancy has been uncomplicated and she has had no invasive testing, no amnio, no ultrasound, and the usual blood testing. She denied having had any pain until the previous week when she developed some pain in her right buttock, which progressed until the day she visited our office. Presently the pain emanates from the right buttock down the leg to the mid-calf. It is worse at night than in the morning. She awakens relatively well each morning and has no difficulty getting out of bed, but by 3 or 4 o'clock in the afternoon her buttock begins to hurt and she progressively gets worse through the evening. The pain is throbbing by 8 o'clock and she finds that she must lie down. On the advice of her midwife she applied ice to the buttocks and low back region three times per day for a period of twenty minutes. The midwife also told her that if the pain becomes extreme and too much to bear she could take one regular strength Tylenol or one "baby" aspirin.

The remainder of Jane's medical history is apparently unremarkable. She wears glasses for an astygmatism since she was 12-years-old, and has worn contact lenses for the last five years until she was pregnant when the extended wear contacts began to bother her during her first trimester. The midwife suggested rather than risk a possible infection that she should just wear regular glasses during the pregnancy. Her mother and father are both living and in good health. Jane has one sibling who is 22 and who has juvenile diabetes which was diagnosed at age 12. Jane reports that her sister has recently graduated from college and will be attending medical school in the fall.

A further review of systems reveals no additional abnormalities nor any other difficulties with any of the following: respiration, breathing, hearing, seeing other than what was already reported; speech, or gait. She reports that she is slightly constipated. She moves her bowels every other day rather than every day when not pregnant. In addition she has an increased frequency of urination, especially in this last month which was checked by the midwife the previous week in a urinalysis to rule out infection. She was found to have none.

Examination

Jane appears to be well-nourished well-developed 25-year-old who presented in the office at 38 weeks pregnant. She weighs 176 lbs. and her height was measured at 5 ft 9 inches (began pregnancy at 145 lbs). Blood pressure 100/68, respiration 29 breaths per minute, pulse 78 beats per minute. Examination of the head and neck was within normal limits. There was no apparent abnormalities seen on fundascopic, otoscopic examinations, no apparent swelling or tenderness was noted. Examination of the throat revealed no apparent swelling or discoloration or lesions present. Auscultation, of the heart and lungs including fremitus was within normal limits. There were no apparent abnormalities in visual and palpable examination of the abdomen and extremities. No edema was present in the feet, hands or legs. No rashes, lesion, abrasion or scars were seen. Leopolds maneuver of the fetus revealed a possible ROP presentation. Orthopedic and neurological examination revealed the following: reflexes: achilles, patellar, biceps, triceps, and brachioradialis to all be +1 (0-2). Orthopedic testing was as follows: Laseque positive right 10 degrees, Hibb negative, Soto Hall negative. Kernigs negative. Pinwheel examination of the lower extremities was the same bilaterally and she did not seem in general to experience a diminished response.

Chiropractic Examination

In addition to the orthopedic and neurological examination performed, static and motion palpation was done on Jane which revealed a loss of range of motion on lateral bending at the waist in addition to waist extension. Both tests began to elicit pain at approximately 20 degrees. Motion palpation of the SI joints revealed a fixation on the right side in a posterior inferior configuration. Static palpation revealed taut and tender fiber at the level of L3 and L5. In addition, pain could be produced upon slight pressure at the sacroiliac joints bilaterally.

Laboratory Tests

A urinalysis was run one week prior to Jane's presentation in the office. She exhibited at that time no signs of the presence of increased WBC's nor the presence of bacteria or elevated levels of protein.

Treatment

Jane was given adjustments at the level of the L5 and the sacroiliac joint. They were performed in the following manner: With the patient prone on a Zenith Hi-lo with the thoraco-lumbar piece extended but not fixed in the open position. The doctor stood on the right side of the patient contacting the right side of the spinous process of L5 with her left fleshy pisiform. Placing the right hand on top of the left hand for stabilization and facing the right side of the patient a thrust was given superiorly to inferiorly, posteriorly to anteriorly, and right to left. (diversifed PR) The sacroiliac joint was adjusted in the following manner. With the patient still prone, the drop mechanism was adjusted to allow for full free fall when a thrust was applied. Once the tension was set in the drop mechanism of the table the doctor then stood on the right side of the table and contacted the lower one third of the right sacroiliac joint with her left fleshy pisiform her fingers on that hand facing the head of the patient. With the right hand placed on top of the left a posterior to anterior inferior to superior thrust was given activating the drop mechanism allowing for the adjustment to be completed. (right PI)

Jane was seen four times over the course of two and a half weeks and the following adjustments administered in a similar manner as above:

Day 3	Right PI/L5 PR
Day 8	Right PI/L3 PR
Day 15	L3 PL/T7 PRS

Discussion

It is clear from Jane's symptomatology that she had what could be considered a sciatic neuralgia of pregnancy. It is important to point out that whenever a pregnant woman presents late in pregnancy with pain, that a differential diagnosis be carefully undertaken so that it is not confused with an appendicitis or some pelvic pain process unrelated to the sciatica. In her case the proper laboratory testing was done to rule out urinary tract infection as well as the proteinuria which may indicate the onset of pre-eclampsia or toxemia. In addition it is interesting to note that Jane's symptomology was clearly defined with the aid of orthopedic testing to be confined to a sciatica which is seen quite often during pregnancy. Research has shown that 50% of all pregnant women experience some type of back pain during pregnancy. With the abdominal presence of the fetus, this causes an increase in the lordosis of the lumbar spine. This causes possible imbrication of the spinous processes of the lumbar spine further altering the intervertebral foramen producing subluxation. This is one of the most common sites of subluxation in pregnancy.

Conclusion

Jane's uncomplicated sciatica resolved after being seen four times over a period of two and a half weeks. She did not have any recurrence of symptomatology until she was 12 weeks postpartum when the pain in the buttocks reappeared. Jane did not have any adjustments after her two and a half weeks of treatment. She immediately however returned when the pain in the buttocks reappeared and now Jane and her two children and husband are patients in the office receiving regular chiropractic care.

A 36-week pregnant woman with pain in her feet

A 27-year-old 36 week pregnant woman presents in the office with pain in her feet. She complains that for the last three weeks her pain has been constant and that she is having trouble walking.

History

Lynda is a 27-year-old 36 week pregnant woman sho presents in the office complaining of pain in both feet. Her neighbor had suggested she go to the chiropractor because maybe the pain was related to the movement of foot bones due to the pregnancy. Lynda reports that her pains are the worst at night and that they are often accompanied by some swelling. When asked further she states that the swelling in her feet has been steady day and night for the last 10 days. She spoke to the nurse at the obstetrician's office five days earlier, and described her feet pain and the nurse told her to soak her feet in epsom salts and to put her feet up as much as possible. It was also recommended that she wear sneakers tightly laced during the day. She tried all of these things but they brought no relief.

This is Lynda's first pregnancy. She reportedly used the pill form of birth control for ten years prior to becoming pregnant. She tried to become pregnant for two years after ceasing the use of birth control. Prior to this time Lynda's pregnancy has been reportedly uneventful. She reported that she gained 41 lbs. during pregnancy which the obstetrician took some exception to. She had a transvaginal ultrasound at 14 weeks which apparently revealed a 14-15 week gestation. In addition she had seen her obstetrician at regular intervals, and had had all the appropriate prenatal testing including a non-stress test, alfa fetoprotein, and urinalysis. A blood count done at 16 weeks revealed a slight anemia for which her obstetrician prescribed ferrous sulfonate. Her last visit to the obstetrician was three weeks earlier and her next visit was scheduled for one week from her presentation in this office.

Her past history revealed allergies to dust mites, dander and strawberries. She received allergy shots from age 8 to age 15. She reportedly had all her childhood illnesses and vaccines. Of note, Lynda had multiple bouts of streptococcal sore throat from age 8 through 11. Each was treated with antibiotics. Her mother and father are living and both are reported to be in excellent health. Her mother (age 50) works full time as an interior designer, and her father (age 49) works full time as the manager of an A&P. Her husband (age 33) of five years is a stock broker.

A review of systems reported no abnormalities. Lynda reported that she did not wear glasses, and denied having any difficulty with urination, bowel movement, gait, respiration or eating or swallowing. She off handedly mentioned that she had some vomiting during the first trimester, which ended at approximately 11 weeks. Since that time she has had no trouble eating or keeping food down. She also had been free from nausea since that time. Other than the pain in her feet, Lynda feels as though she has had a normal pregnancy.

Examination

Examination of Lynda revealed a slightly built 27-year-old 36 week pregnant woman weighing 191 pounds and measuring 5 ft 5 inches tall. Her vital signs were as follows: BP 140/85, Respiration 29 breaths per minute regular and very shallow, Pulse 88 beats per minute, strong and regular. Her temperature was 98.2. A repeat blood pressure done on the right arm was 138/84. Examination of the head and neck including fundascopic, and ottoscopic examination was within normal limits. No apparent swelling, abrasions, lesions or scars were noted. Examination of the oral cavity was within normal limits. All cranial nerve function appeared to be within normal limits except her jaw jerk reflex which appeared to be +2 (0-2). Ausculation of the heart, and lung fields including fremitus appeared to be within normal limits. Leopolds maneuver revealed a probably LOA presentation (with head down and occiput toward the anterior). Orthopedic examination was within normal limits including laseque, Braggards, contralateral laseque, Hibb, and Soto Hall. Reflexes were as follows: Achilles right +2, left +1 (0-2). Patellar right +1, left +1, Brachioradilais, biceps, and triceps all +1 bilaterally. Examination of the feet and hands revealed slight swelling of the hands and moderate to severe swelling of the feet and ankles. On the left, the swelling reached to the mid-calf region. When the edema was pushed in, small pit-like areas formed around the examiner's thumb. The arches on both feet had become completely obiterated and fallen in each foot.

Discussion

At this juncture, it is most important to stop and look at the possible differential diagnoses that Lynda could be experiencing. While it would be simple to characterize this as simply fallen arches of pregnancy with complicating edema, there appears to be a larger picture developing. Most all pregnant women experience a decrease in the level of their blood pressure. This enables their bodies to accommodate for the changes in blood volume and heart stoke volume, without risking the possibility of a stroke. The decrease in peripheral resistance created by the level of hormones in their systems only adds to their ability to withstand tremendous increases in pressure during labor and delivery. In Lynda's case her blood pressure has become slightly elevated, which becomes something of a concern. Coupled with the presence of edema which in and of itself is not of concern, yet it is of the "pitting" quality in Lynda, and more importantly coupled with some slight hyper-reflexia, must lead the doctor to consider immediately the presence of pre-eclampsia and or full toxemia. At this point it is important to send the woman to her pregnancy care-giver with the positive findings. At this point a urinalysis needs to be performed to look for the presence of protein. If indeed protein is present in the urine, toxemia can be confirmed. It is however at this time not appropriate to allow the patient to wait a week for her regular appointment. The doctor must call the obstetrician or midwife and inform her or him of the presence of hyper-reflexia and the other findings including the increase in blood pressure.

Conclusion

Upon further examination of the patient by the obstetrician she was concluded to have pre-eclampsia, and was immediately asked to remain at home on bed rest and reduce her fluid intake. After two weeks of being stable without another increase in the blood pressure, Lynda had an induced labor and gave birth after 18 hours of labor to a healthy young girl. She returned postpartum to the office for follow-up work on her feet and her back as she developed sciatica during the birth. ■

11 Childbirth Education and the Chiropractor

One of the most important aspects of the care of the pregnant woman is childbirth education. In the past, childbirth education was the domain of the obstetrician and the old "wives tales" that were handed down mother to daughter. The 1990s is known as the age of information and patients are becoming educated consumers. This is especially true in the realm of childbirth. Twenty-five years ago any type of childbirth education was unheard of, in today's society most pregnant women attend some type of childbirth class whether they be purely educational or exercise oriented.

One of the most protective mechanisms that an individual can employ is education. The pregnant woman can help to maintain the integrity of the birth process by becoming as educated as possible and to actively participate in that process. In addition, gone are the days where the father remains in the waiting room as the baby is born, leaving the entire process to the doctors and nurses without his active participation. Now childbirth education routinely involves both parents and rightly so.

The midwife

At one time, childbirth was the domain of the local midwife. Medically untrained but trained usually through experience, she usually delivered all the children within a given town or regional area. It was a "profession" handed down, mother to daughter, grandmother to granddaughter, often the only option in childbirth. Once medicine began to gain hold of all medical procedures, and with the advent of sterile techniques, childbirth gradually became the domain of the medical doctors and the hospital. The birthing of children went from a female oriented profession to a male oriented one. So in addition to the change of venue from the home to the hospital, the practice of obstetrics changed from one group of individuals to another. In addition to the sterile techniques that began to be employed during childbirth, many techniques of convenience began to emerge in the practice of obstetrics which were not always in the best interest of the mother or the newborn child. These changes became so extreme that in the 1950's and 60's and into the 70's the obstetric practitioner began to see the domain of childbirth, and the challenge of practice begin to change. Women were beginning to question birth outcomes and the incidence of liability began to rise. Medicine in general by this time had become more and more impersonal. One of the most personal experiences in a woman's life is her birthing experience, and with impersonalization of medicine, and a poor birth outcome, the incidence of liability rose to tremendous proportions in the mid 1980's.

At this same time a new type of practitioner began to emerge, the Certified Nurse Midwife. The Certified Nurse Midwife is an RN who has at least three years postgraduate experience in gynecology, labor, and delivery. This new type of practitioner delivers an obstetrical care that is more encompassing and more personal than that of the obstetrician. The Midwife is filling a place in the healthcare system that has been desperately needed for many years. Without the tremendous liability issues due to the fact that they perform no surgery (no C-sections), the CNM is able to spend more time with each patient, and is better able to give bedside care and support during labor and delivery which are so necessary.

In a complicated pregnancy which may require intervention it is essential to have present the appropriate practitioner who can perform a C-section if necessary. The CNM however serves a special purpose in the process of labor and delivery that is very important. All the major University Hospitals in New York City have CNMs on staff, and some CNMs even maintain private practices in hospitals.

I am often asked about the lay Midwife. Again, the level of competency that is proportional to the level of experience of the CNM holds true for the lay midwife. Since there is no standard by which the lay midwife is measured, it is more difficult to assess the skill and competency of the lay midwife. Whereas the CNM must undergo rigorous testing procedures and state licensing examinations, the lay midwife can practice in a purely uncontrolled environment.

Many women desire to have a birth at home, and in most states this is either illegal or very difficult due to the alternative backup needed should medical intervention be necessary. In this case, if the parents' wish to have a home birth they must do so with a lay midwife. This should only be undertaken when it is a low-risk childbirth as there is no evidence that a hospital is a better setting for a low-risk child birth than the home. Careful attention should be paid however, to the qualifications and experience of the lay midwife, and what parameters are likely to be followed in the event of an emergency.

Labor support doulas

A doula is literally defined as a woman who serves women, but in today's vernacular it has come to mean a woman who supports and cares for another woman during labor, birth and the postpartum. According to Teresa Goetz, C.C.E one of the leading authorities on doulas and labor support, and owner of Birth Renaissance a complete facility given to the education of the pregnant woman, and friend to chiropractic: "For most of history, women birthed with the support and presence of other women. Laboring women benefited from the wisdom and shared experience of these attendants. As birth moved into the hospital, the womanly ways of birth disappeared, and women themselves were increasingly removed from the birth experience through the use of narcotics and isolation. Nurturing and encouragement were replaced with medical management."

Most labor support doulas have formal training, and some are either part of the childbirth education network, and others are women who have studied childbirth. The labor support doula can help where the father or partner can not. Whether it be a breathing exercise, or a helpful hint with respect to decreasing pain during labor, or even just an encouraging word, the doula fills a special place during the birth. It has also been shown that the presence of a labor support doula can alter the birth outcome and state of the mother.

International Childbirth Education Association

One of the finest organizations to be involved in childbirth education is the International Childbirth Education Association (ICEA). Their goal is contained in their motto: "Freedom of Choice Through Knowledge of Alternatives." Each ICEA practitioner teaches childbirth classes from this perspective. This is a worldwide organization which teaches parents about pregnancy and the process of childbirth from a natural alternative and scientific basis. Using scientific data, they critically examine the medical norms for childbirth and teach their efficacy and the efficacy of their alternatives. The author recommends that doctors encourage all new parents to take childbirth classes from a Certified Childbirth Educator (CCE) so they will receive correct information about the process of childbirth, and the alternatives.

Chiropractic

The chiropractor serves a special need in the case of the pregnant woman. The obstetrician/midwife are reluctant to assume responsibility for an illness that lies beyond the scope of obstetrics or gynecology. The general practitioner or family practitioner is reluctant to prescribe any type of medicine or care for the woman who is ill, and her condition is dominated by the pregnancy and in their eyes falls within the scope of the practitioner who is caring for the pregnancy. This leaves the pregnant woman at times in a quandary and basically without care for conditions unrelated to her pregnancy. Chiropractors know that restoring optimal nerve function can often times enable the body to heal itself. Therefore, chiropractic is an invaluable asset to the pregnant woman, not only in terms of the pregnancy, but in terms of overall health.

Chiropractors are in a wonderful position to help with the care of the pregnant woman. The physiology of pregnancy lends itself to subluxative changes and subsequent correction by the chiropractor. It is clear that most if not all of the orthopedic and neurological conditions of pregnancy are a result of physiologically induced subluxation which can be corrected by chiropractic care. The pregnant woman needs chiropractic care and I firmly believe that the chiropractor can help the pregnant woman and the children she bears. ■

REFERENCES

Adjusting the Pregnant Woman

Fallon JM: Chiropractic and pregnancy, Articles on Pediatrics Vol I, International Review of Chiropractic, 1994

Fallon JM: Orthopedic and neurological conditions of pregnancy, Multimedia Presentation, 1990

Fallon JM: Orthopedic and neurological conditions of pregnancy and chiropractic management of care, Articles on Pediatrics Vol II, International Review of Chiropractic, 1994

Fallon JM: The biomechanical and hormonal considerations of pregnancy as they relate to chiropractic care, Multimedia presentation 1989, 1993

Bibliography

EFFECTS OF THERAPEUTIC DRUGS:

Aase JM: Anticonvulsant drugs and congenital abnormalities. Amer J Disease of Children 127:758, 1974

Anderson RC: Cardiac defects in children of mothers receiving anticonvulsant therapy during pregnancy. J of Pediatrics, 89:318, 1976

Callaghan N, Garrett A, Goggin T: Withdrawal of anticonvulsant drugs in patients free of seizures for two years. N Engl J Med, 318:942 1988

Diggory PLC, Tomkinson JS: Nausea and Vomiting in pregnancy: A trial of Meclizine dihydrochloride with and without pyridoxine Lancet, 2:370, 1962

Hartz SC, Heinonen OP, Shapiro S, et.al.: Antenatal exposure to meprobamate and chlordiazepoxide in relation to malformation, mental development, and childhood mortality. N Engl J Med, 292:726 1975

Laegreid L, Olegard R, Wahlstrom J et.al.: Abnormalities in children exposed to benzodiazepines in utero. Lancet, 1:108,1987

Mujtaba Q, Burrow GN: Treatment of Hyperthyroidism in pregnancy with propylthiouricil and Methimazole. Obstet Gynecol, 46:282, 1975

Nakane Y, Okuma T, Takahashi R, et.al.: Multi institutional study on the teratogenicity and fetal toxicity of antiepileptic drugs: A report of a collaborative study group in Japan. Epilepsia, 21:663, 1980

Rumeau-Rouquette C, Goujard J, Huel G: Possible teratogenic effect of phenothiazines in human beings. Teratology, 15:57 1977

Safra MJ, Oakly GP: Association between cleft lip with or without cleft palate and prenatal exposure to diazepam. Lancet, 2:478 1975

ECTOPIC PREGNANCY

Barnes AB, Wennberg CN, Barnes BA: Ectopic Pregnancy: Incidence and review of determinant factors. Obstet Gynecol Surv, 38:345 1983

Dorfman SF: Deaths from ectopic pregnancy, United States 1979 to 1980. Obstet Gynecol, 62:334, 1983

Loffer FD: Current concepts ion the management of ectopic pregnancies. J Reprod Med, 31:73 1986

ANATOMY & PHYSIOLOGY

Austin CR: Fertilization. Prentice-Hall, Englewood Cliffs, N.J., 1965

Austin CR: Sperm maturation in the male and female genital tracts. In Metz CB.Monray A (eds): Biology of Fertilization, Volume 2, Academic Press, New York, 1985

Braude P, Bolton V, Moore S: Human gene expression first occurs between the four- and eight-cell stages of the preimplantation development. Nature, 332:459, 1988

Braunstein GD, Rasor JL, Engvall E, et.al.: Interrelationships of human chorionic gonadatropin, human placental lactogen and pregnancy-specific glycoprotein throughout normal human gestation. Am J Obstet Gynecol, 138:1205 1980

Csapo AL, Pulkkinen MO: Indispensability of the human corpus luteum in the maintenance of early pregnancy luteectomy evidence. Obstet Gynecol Surv, 33:69 1978

Eastman NJ, Hellman LM: Williams Obstetrics, 13th ed. Appleton-Century-Crofts, New York, 1966

Fallon JM: Orthopedic and neurological conditions of pregnancy, Multimedia Presentation, 1990

Fallon JM: The biomechanical and hormonal considerations of pregnancy as they relate to chiropractic care, Multimedia presentation 1989, 1993

Gill TJ III, Immunity and Pregnancy. CRC Crit Rev Immunol, 5:201, 1985

Grant JCB: An Atlas of the Human Body. 7th ed. Williams and Wilkins, Baltimore, 1978

Hearn JP: The embryo-maternal dialogue during early pregnancy in primates. J Reprod Fertil, 76:809, 1986

Hunziker RD, Wegmann TG, Placental immunoregulation. CRC Crit Rev Immunol, 6:245 1987

Knobil E, Neill J (eds): The Physiology of Reproduction, Raven Press, New York, 1988

Lenton EA, Neal LM, Sulaiman R: Plasma concentrations of human chorionic gonadatropin from the time of implantation until the second week of pregnancy. Fertil Steril, 37:773 1982

Ludwig H, Metzer H, The Human Female Reproductive Tract. A Scanning Electron Microscope Atlas, Springer-Verlag, Heidelberg, 1976

McMullen M: Assessing cervical subluxations in infants under six months of age. Articles on Pediatrics Vol I. International Review of Chiropractic, 1994

Moore KL: The Developing Human, 4th ed. Philadelphia, WB Saunders, 1988

Pauerstein CJ, Hodgson BJ, Kramen MA: The anatomy and physiology of the oviduct. Obstet Gynecol Ann, 3:317 1974

Scott JR., DiSaia PJ, Hammond CB., Spellacy WN. Danforth's Obstetrics and Gynecology 6th ed. J.B. Lippincott Company, Philadelphia, 1990

Sholls HT, Orsini MW, Hitchins DJ: Estrogen synthesis and metabolism in the hamster blastocyst, uterus and liver near the time of implantation. J Steroid Biochem, 19:1153 1983

Ulfelder H: Mechanism of pelvic support in women. Am J of Obstet Gynecol, 72:856, 1956

Wynn RM(ed) Cellular Biology of the Uterus, Appleton-Century-Crofts, New York, 1967

NEUROMUSCULAR SKELETAL SYSTEM

Adour KK: The bell tolls for decompression? N Engl J Med, 292:748, 1975

Aminoff MJ: Neurological disorders and pregnancy. Am J Obstet Gynecol, 132:325,1978

Bell C: The Nervous System of the Human Body. Longman Rees, Orme, Brown, and Green. London, 1830

Berg G, Hammer M, Moller-Nielson J, et.al.: Low back pain during pregnancy. Obstet and Gynecol, 72:71

Berkwitz NJ and Lufkin NH: Toxic neuronitis of pregnancy: A clinicopathological report. Surg, Gynecol and Obstet, 54:743, 1932

Benson RC, Inman VT: Brachialgia statica dysesthetica in pregnancy. Western Journal of Surgery, 64:115, 1956

Brown JT and McDougall A: Traumatic maternal birth palsy, J Obstet and Gynecol of the British Empire, 64:431

Cole JT: Maternal obstetric paralysis, Amer J Obstet and Gynecol, 52:386

Ecker AD and Woltman HW: Meralgia Parestetica: A report of one hundred and fifty cases, J Amer Med Assoc, 110:1650, 1938

Eckman-Ordeberg G, Salgeback S, Ordeberg G: Carpal Tunnel Syndrome in pregnancy. A prospective study. Acta Obstet Gynecol Scand, 66:233, 1987

Fallon JM: Orthopedic and neurological conditions of pregnancy and chiropractic management of care, Articles on Pediatrics Vol II, International Review of Chiropractic, 1994

Fallon JM: Orthopedic and neurological conditions of pregnancy, Multimedia Presentation, 1990, 1994

Fallon JM: The biomechanical and hormonal considerations of pregnancy as they relate to chiropractic care, Multimedia presentation 1989, 1993, 1994

Fisher AP, Hanna M: Transcutaneous nerve stimulation in meralgia parestetica of pregnancy, British J of Ob Gyn, 94:603, 1987

Font AT, Hankin RS: Pregnancy outcomes after now catastrophic maternal trauma during pregnancy. Obstet Gynecol, 35:912, 1970

Forster JB: Hydrocortisone and the carpal tunnel syndrome, Lancet, 1:456, 1960

Head HB, Welsh JS, Mussey E et.al.: Cyclic sciatica: Report of case with introduction of a new surgical sign. J Am Med Assoc, 180:521, 1962

Hamlin E, Lehman RAW: Carpal Tunnel Syndrome, New Engl J Med, 276:849, 1967

Jones MW, Berry K: Chronic relapsing polyneuritis associated with pregnancy, Transactions of the Obstetrical Society of London, 9:12, 1981

Ironside R: Neuritis complicating Pregnancy, Proceedings of the Royal Society of Medicine, 32:588, 1939

King G, Ride LT: The relation of vitamin B1 deficiency to pregnancy toxemias. J of Obstet Gynecol of British Empire, 52:130, 1945

McMullen M: Assessing cervical subluxations in infants under six months of age. Articles on Pediatrics Vol I. International Review of Chiropractic, 1994

McMullen M: Handicapped children and chiropractic care (Part I, II). Articles on Pediatrics Vol 1. International Review of Chiropractic, 1994

O'Connell JEA: Lumbar Disc Protrusion in Pregnancy. J of Neurology, Neurosurgery and Psychiatry, 23:138, 1960

Prineas J: Peripheral nerve changes in thiamine-deficient rats. Archives of Neurology, 23:541, 1970

Sands RX: Bachache of pregnancy: a method of treatment. Obstet Gynecol, 12:670, 1958

Sommerville BW: A study of migraines in pregnancy. Neurology, 22:824, 1972

Strauss MB, McDonald WJ: Polyneuritis of pregnancy: A dietary deficiency disorder. J Amer Med Assoc, 100:1320, 1933

Robinson JR, Pou JW: Bell's Palsy: A predisposition of pregnant women. Archives of Otolaryngology, 95:125, 1972

Romberg MH: Diseases of the Nervous System Vol II, Sydenham Society, London, 1851

Urist MR: Obstetric fracture-dislocation of the pelvis: Report of a case with injury to the lumbosacral trunk and first sacral nerve roots. J Amer Med Assoc, 152:127, 1953

ANESTHESIA DURING BIRTH

Alpher MH: Toxicity of local anesthetics. New Eng J Med, 295:1432, 1976

Atrash HK, Koonin LM, Lawson HW, Franks AL, Smith JC: Maternal Mortality in the United States, 1979-1986. Obstet Gynecol, 76:1055, 1990

Friedman JM: Teratogen update: Anesthetic agents. Teratology 37:69, 1988

Hellman K: Epidural anaesthesia in obstetrics. Canadian Anaesthetics Society Journal, 12:398, 1965

Lamaze F: Painless Childbirth: Psychoprophylactic Method. Henry Regnery, Chicago, 1970

Potts CR, Ullery JC: Maternal and fetal effects of obstetric anesthesia: Intravenous use of promethazine and meperidine. Am J Obstet Gynecol, 81:1253, 1961

Wagman IH, deJong RN, Prince DA: Effects of lidocaine on the central nervous system, Anesthes, 28:155, 1967

SYSTEMIC CHANGES DURING PREGNANCY

Anderson LL: Regulation of relaxin secretion and it's role in pregnancy. Adv Exp Med Biol, 219:421, 1987

Baird JD: Some Aspects of the metabolic and hormonal adaptation to pregnancy. Acta Endocrinol (suppl) (Copenh), 277:11, 1986

Brody SA, Ueland K (eds): Endocrine Disorders in Pregnancy, Appleton & Lange, Norwalk, 1989

Chesley LC, Sibai BM: Blood pressure in the midtrimester and future pre-eclampsia. Am J Obstet Gynecol, 157:1258, 1987

Davison JM: Kidney function in pregnant women. Am J Kidney Dis, 9:265, 1987

DeSwiet M: The respiratory system. In Hytten FE, Chanberlain G(eds): Clinical Physiology in Obstetrics, 2nd ed. Oxford, Blackwell, 1991

Douvas SG, Meeks GR, Phillips JC, et.al.: Liver disease in pregnancy. Obstet Gynecol Surv, 38:531, 1983

Easterling TR, Schumucker BC, Benedetti TJ: The haemodynamic effects of orthostatic stress during pregnancy. Obstet Gynecol, 72:550, 1988

Fallon JM: Orthopedic and neurological conditions of pregnancy, Multimedia Presentation, 1990

Fallon JM: The biomechanical and hormonal considerations of pregnancy as they relate to chiropractic care, Multimedia presentation 1989, 1993

Gant NF, Whalley PJ, Everett RB, et.al.: Control of vascular reactivity in pregnancy. Am. J. Kidney Disease, 9:303, 1987

Grant JCB: An Atlas of the Human Body. 7th ed. Williams and Wilkins, Baltimore, 1978

Klein EA: Urologic problems in pregnancy: A review. Obstet Gyecol Surv, 39:605, 1984

Lind T: Metabolic changes in pregnancy relevant to diabetes mellitus. Postgrad Med J, 55:353, 1979

Macfie AG, Magides AP, et. al.: Gastric emptying in pregnancy. Br J Anaesth, 67:54, 1991

Metcalfe J, McAnulty JH, Ueland K: Burwell and Metcalfe's Heart Disease in Pregnancy: Physiology and Management. Little, Brown, Boston, 1986

Milne JS, Howie AD, Pack AI: Dyspnoea during normal pregnancy. Br. J Obstet Gynaecol, 85:260, 1978

Pritchard JA, Scott DE: Iron stores of normal adults and their replenishment with oral iron therapy. JAMA, 190:897, 1964

Smout CFV, Jacoby F, Lillie EW: Gynecological and Obstetrical Anatomy. Williams and Wilkins, Baltimore, 1969

LYME DISEASE

Mikkelsen AL, Palle C: Lyme disease during pregnancy. Avcta Obstetrica et Gynecologia Scandinavica, 66:477, 1983

Pacher AR, Steere AC: The triad of neurological manifestations of Lyme disease. Neurology, 35:47, 1986

Reik, SteereAC, Bartenhagen NH et.al.: Neurological abnormalities of Lyme disease without erythema chronicum migrans. Amer J of Medicine, 81:73, 1986

MALPRESENTATION

Amirikia H, Zarewych B, Evans TN: Cesarean section: A 15 year review of changing incidence, indications and risks. Am J Obstet Gynecol, 140:81, 1981

Bird GC: The use of the vacuum extractor. Clin Obstet Gynecol, 9:641, 1982

Collea JV, Rabin SC, Weghorst GR, et al: The randomized management of term frank breech presentations: Vaginal delivery vs cesarean section. Am J Obstet Gynecol, 131:186, 1978

Cruikshank DP, White CA: Obstetric malpresentations: Twenty years experience. Am J Obst Gynecol, 116:1097, 1973

Dyson DC, Mellder PD, Armstrong MA: Management of prolonged pregnancy: Induction of labor versus antepartum fetal testing. Am J Obstet Gynecol, 156:928, 1987

Levine MG, Holroyde J, Woods JR, et al. Birth trauma: Incidence and predisposing factors. Obstet Gynecol, 63:792, 1984

McMullen M: Assessing cervical subluxations in infants under six months of age. Articles on Pediatrics Vol I, International Review of Chiropractic, 1994

McMullen M: Handicapped children and chiropractic care (Part I & II). Articles on Pediatrics Vol 1, International Review of Chiropractic, 1994

Ryden G: Vacuum extraction or forceps? (Editorial) Br Med J, 292:75 1986

Taffel SM, Placek PJ, Liss T: Trends in the United States cesarean section rate and reasons for the 1980-85 rise. Am J Pub Health, 77:955, 1987

BREAST CANCER

Harris JR, Rechet A, Connally et al: Conservative surgery and radiotherapy for early breast cancer. Cancer, 66:15427, 1990

Huguley CM Jr., Brown RL: The value of breast self-examination. Cancer, 47:989, 1990

OPERATIVE BIRTH

Amirika H, Zarewych B, Evans TN: Cesarean section: A 15 year review of changing incidence, indications and risks. Am J Obstet Gynecol, 140:81, 1987

Bird GC: The use of the vacuum extractor. Clin Obstet Gynecol, 9:641,1982

Broekhuizen FF, Washington JM, Johnson F, Hamilton PR: Vacuum extraction versus forceps delivery: Indications and complications, 1979 to 1984. Ob Gynecol, 69:338, 1987

Cesarean Childbirth: Report of a Concensus Development Conference. US Dept. of Health and Human Services. Bethesda MD, NIH Publication No. 82-2067, Oct 1981

Dyson DC, Mellder PD, Armstrong MA: Management of prolonged pregnancy: Induction of labor versus antepartum fetal testing. Am J Obstet Gynecol, 156:928, 1987

Gibbs RS, Jones PM, Wilder CJT: Internal fetal monitoring and maternal infection following cesarean section. Obstet Gynecol, 52:193, 1978

Ryden G: Vacuum extraction or forceps? (Editorial) Br Med J, 292:75 1986

Taffel SM, Placek PJ, Liss T: Trends in the United States cesarean section rate and reasons for the 1980-85 rise. Am J Pub Health, 77:955, 1987

BREAST FEEDING

Anath J: Side effects in the neonate from psychotropic agents: excretion through breast feeding. Am J Psychiatry, 135:801, 1987

Behrem RE (ed.): Neonatal-perinatal Medicine (2nd ed.) C.V. Mosby, St. Louis, 1977

Catz CS, Yaffee SJ: Environmental factors: Phamacology in Prevention of Embryonic fetal and Perinatal Disease, Chapter 6. Washington: U.S. Govt Printing Office

Knowles JA: Excretion of drugs in milk: A review. J of Pediatrics, 66: 1068, 1965

TOXEMIA

Beck DW, Menezes AH: Intracerebral hemorrhage in the patient with eclampsia. J of Am Med Ass, 246:1442, 1981

Chesley LC: The origin of the word 'eclampsia'. Obstet and Gynecol, 39:802, 1972

Gaitz JP, Bamford CR: unusual computed tomographic scan in eclampsia. Archives of Neurology, 39:66 1982

Gowers WR: A Manual of Diseases of the Nervous System. Blakiston Son & Co. Philadelphia, 1888.

Sheehan HL, Lynch JB: Pathology of Toxemia of Pregnancy. Williams and Wilkins, Baltimore, 1973.

NEONATE

Anthony CL, Arnon R, Fitch CW: Pediatric Cardiology, Medical Outline Series. Medical Examination Publishing Co, Flushing N.Y., 1979

Barness LA: Manual of Pediatric Physical Diagnosis (4th ed.) Year Book Med, Chicago, 1972

Behrem RE (ed.): Neonatal-Perinatal Medicine (2nd ed), C.V. Mosby, St. Louis, 1977

Coleman SS: Congenital dysplasia and dislocation of the hip. C.V. Mosby Co., St. Louis, 1978

Cox D: The condyle subluxation in infants, Articles on Pediatrics, International Review of Chiropractic, Vol II, 1994

Kent C: An overview of pediatric radiology, Articles on Pediatrics Vol I, International Review of Chiropractic, 1994

Lovell WW, Winter RB: Pediatric Orthopaedics. J.B. Lippincott Co, Philadelphia, 1978

McMullen M: Assessing cervical subluxations in infants under six months of age. Articles on Pediatrics Vol I . International Review of Chiropractic, 1994

McMullen M: Handicapped children and chiropractic care (Part I, II). Articles on Pediatrics Vol 1. International Review of Chiropractic, 1994

Mellott S: Pediatric radiology, Articles on Pediatrics Vol II, International Review of Chiropractic, 1994

Roberts NK, Gelband H: Cardiac Arrhythmias in the neonate infant and child. Appleton-Century-Crofts, New York, 1977

Scarpelli EM, Auld PAM: Pulmonary Physiology of the Fetus Newborn and Child. Lea & Febiger, Philadelphia, 1975

ADJUSTING THE PREGNANT WOMAN

DeBoer KF, Harmon RO, Savoie, Tuttle CD: Inter and intra-examiner reliability of leg length differential measurement: a preliminary study. J Manip Physiolog Ther, 6:61, 1983

Fallon JM: Chiropractic and Pregnancy, Articles on Pediatrics Vol I, International Review of Chiropractic, 1994

Fallon JM: Orthopedic and neurological conditions of pregnancy, Multimedia Presentation, 1990

Fallon JM: Orthopedic and neurological conditions of pregnancy and chiropractic management of care, Articles on Pediatrics Vol II, International Review of Chiropractic, 1994

Fallon JM: The biomechanical and hormonal considerations of pregnancy as they relate to chiropractic care, Multimedia presentation 1989, 1993

Finneson BE (ed): Low Back Pain. Lippincott, Philadelphia, 1980

Grostic J: Some observations on computer-aided x-ray analysis. Int Rev Chiropractic, 33:38, 1979

Haldeman S: Spinal Manipulative Therapy. Clin Orthop, 179:62, 1983

Hamlin E, Lehman RAW: Carpal Tunnel Syndrome, New Engl J Med, 276:849, 1967

Ironside R: Neuritis complicating pregnancy, Proceedings of the Royal Society of Medicine, 32:588, 1939

Palmer DD: The Science, Art and Philosophy of Chiropractic, Portland Printing House, Portland, 1910

Palmer MH: Chiropractic Anatomy Vol IX, Palmer College of Chiropractic, Davenport, 1929

Ulfelder H: Mechanism of pelvic support in women. Am J of Obstet Gynecol, 72:856, 1956

ORTHOPEDIC/ NEUROLOGICAL CONDITIONS

Berg G, Hammar M, Moller-Nielsen J et al: Low back pain during pregnancy. Obstet and Gynecol, 72:71, 1988

Cohen BA, London RS, Goldstein PJ: Myastenia gravis and preeclampsia. Obstet and Gynecol, 48:35s, 1976

Davis FA: Impairment of repetitive impulse conduction in experimentally demyelinated and pressure injured nerves. J Neurol Neurosurg, Psychiatry, 39:443, 1972

Dalessio DJ: Classification and treatment of headache during pregnancy. Clinical Neuropharmocology, 9:121, 1986

Fallon JM: Orthopedic and neurological conditions of pregnancy, Multimedia Presentation, 1990

Fallon JM: The biomechanical and hormonal considerations of pregnancy as they relate to chiropractic care, Multimedia presentation 1989, 1993

Farfan HF: Mechanical Disorders of the Low Back, Lea & Febiger, Philadelphia, 1973

Gelb HGL: Clinical Management of Head, Neck and TMJ Pain and Dysfunction. Saunders, Philadelphia, 1977

Gilliatt RW: The cause of nerve damage in acute compression. Trans Am Neurol Assoc, 99:71, 1974

Haldemen S (ed): Modern Developments in the Principles and Practice of Chiropractic, Appleton-Century-Crofts, New York, 1980

Haldeman S: Interactions between the somatic and visceral nervous systems. ACA J Chiropractic, 5:57, 1971.

Hammar M, Larsson L, Tegler L: Calcium treatment of leg cramps in pregnancy. Acta Obstetrica et Gynecologia Scandinavica, 60:345, 1981

Homewood AE: The Neurodynamics of the Vertebral Subluxation. Valkyrie Press, St. Petersburg, 1979

Janse JH, Wells BF, et al: Chiropractic Principles and Technic, National College of Chiropractic, Chicago, 1947

Kopell HP: Help For Your Aching Back, Grosset & Dunlap, New York, 1969

LaBan MM, Perrin JCS, Latimer FR: Pregnancy and the herniated lumbar disc. Archives of Phy. Med and Rehabil, 64:320, 1983

Leach RA: The Chiropractic Theories, Williams & Wilkins, Baltimore, 1986

Lind GAM: Auto-Traction Treatment of Low Back Pain and Sciatica. Linkoping, Sweden, 1974

Lord JW Jr, Rosalie LM: Neurovascular Compression Syndromes of the Upper Extremity. Clin Symp, 23:2, 1971

Lowe TW, Weinreb J, Santos-Ramos R et al: Magnetic resonance imaging in human pregnancy. Obstet and Gynecol, 66:629, 1985

Lusted LB, Leats TE: Atlas of Roentgenographic Measurement. (2nd ed.) Chicago Yearbook, Chicago, 1967

MacGibbon B, Farfan HF: Are all lumbar spines the same- radiological survey. Spine 4:258, 1979

Oswald I: Sudden body jerks on falling asleep. Brain, 82:92, 1959

Pacher AR, Steere AC: The triad of neurological manifestations of Lyme disease. Neurology, 35:47, 1986

Palmateer DC: Greater occipital-trigeminal syndrome. J Clin Chiropractic (arch ed.) Winter, 1972

Poser S, Poser W: Multiple sclerosis and gestatation. Neurology, 33:1422, 1983

Putti V: New conceptions in the pathogenesis of sciatic pain, Lancet, 2:53, 1927

Rainer GW, Mayer J, Sadler TR, Dirks D: Effects of graded compression on nerve conduction velocity. Arch Surg, 107:719, 1973

Reik L, Steere AC, Bartenhagen NH et al: Neurological abnormalities of Lyme disease without erythema chronicum migrans. Amer J of Medicine, 81:73, 1986

Schmorl G, Junghanns H: The Human Spine in Health and Disease (2nd ed.) Grune & Stratton, New York, 1971

Suh CH: Computer Aided Design Mechanisms. University of Colorado, Boulder, 1975

Wall PD, Waxman S, Basbaum AI: Ongoing activity in peripheral nerve: Injury discharge. Exp Neurol, 45:576, 1974

Wright DO, Patel MK: Focal migraine and pregnancy. British Med Journal, 293:1557, 1986

POST PARTUM DEPRESSION

Fondeur M, Vixsen C, Triebel WA et al: Postpartum mental illness: A controlled study. Archives of Neurology and Psychiatry, 77:503, 1957

Lloyd JH: Puerpural insanity and the insanity of pregnancy and lactation. In A System of Obstetrics. Vol 2, Lea Brothers, Philadelphia, 1889

Robin AA: The psychological changes of normal parturition. Psychiatric Quarterly, 36:129, 1962

Zilborg G: Depressive reactions related to parenthood. American J of Psychiatry, 10:927, 1931

CONGENITAL ABNORMALITIES

Aase JM: Anticonvulsant drugs and congenital abnormalities. Amer J Disease of Children, 127:758, 1974

Anderson RC: Cardiac defects in children of mothers receiving anticonvulsant therapy during pregnancy. J of Pediatrics, 89:318, 1976

Bjeredal T: Epilepsy, Pregnancy and the Child. Raven Press, New York, 1982

Dansky LV, Andermann E, Rosenblatt D et al: Anticonvulsants, folate levels, and pregnancy outcome: A prospective study. Annals of Neurology, 21:176, 1987

McMullen M: Assessing cervical subluxations in infants under six months of age. Articles on Pediatrics Vol I . International Review of Chiropractic, 1994

McMullen M: Handicapped children and chiropractic care (Part I & II). Articles on Pediatrics Vol 1. International Review of Chiropractic, 1994

HORMONES OF PREGNANCY

Baird DT: Preface. In Baird DT, Michie EA (eds.): Mechanisms of Menstrual Bleeding. Raven Press, New York, 1985

Bradbury JT, Brown WE, Guay LA: Maintenance of the corpus luteum and physiological action of progesterone. Recent Prog Horm Res, 5:151, 1950

Braunstein GD, Rasor JL, Engvall E, et al: Interrelationships of human chorionic gonadatropin, human placental lactogen and pregnancy-specific glycoprotein throughout normal human gestation. Am J Obstet Gynecol, 138:1205 1980

Cassmer O: Hormone production of the isolated human placenta. Acta Endocrinol, 32 (suppl):45, 1959

Csapo AL, Pulkkinen MO: Indispensability of the human corpus luteum in the maintenance of early pregnancy luteectomy evidence. Obstet Gynecol Surv, 33:69 1978

Eastman NJ, Hellman LM: Williams Obstetrics, 13th ed. Appleton-Century-Crofts, New York, 1966

Fallon JM: Orthopedic and neurological conditions of pregnancy, Multimedia Presentation, 1990, 1994

Fallon JM: The biomechanical and hormonal considerations of pregnancy as they relate to chiropractic care, Multimedia presentation 1989, 1993, 1994

Gill TJ III, Immunity and Pregnancy. CRC Crit Rev Immunol, 5:201, 1985

Hearn JP: The embryo-maternal dialogue during early pregnancy in primates. J Reprod Fertil, 76:809, 1986

Hunziker RD, Wegmann TG, Placental immunoregulation. CRC Crit Rev Immunol, 6:245 1987

Khodr GS, Siler-Khodr TM: Placental lutenizing hormone-releasing factor and its synthesis. Science, 207:315, 1980

Knobil E, Neill J (eds): The Physiology of Reproduction, Raven Press, New York, 1988

Lenton EA, Neal LM, Sulaiman R: Plasma concentrations of human chorionic gonadatropin from the time of implantation until the second week of pregnancy. Fertil Steril, 37:773 1982

Potter EL, Craig JM: Pathology of the fetus and infant. Chicago, Year Book, 1975

Smout CFV, Jacoby F, Lillie EW: Gynecological and Obstetrical Anatomy. Williams and Wilkins, Baltimore, 1969

PRENATAL TESTING

American College of Obstetricians and Gynecologists (ACOG): Technical Bulletin No.108. Antenatal diagnosis of genetic disorders. Washington, D.C. ACOG Meeting, 1987

Cackle H, Wald NJ, Bankau G. et. al.: biochemical screening for Downs syndrome. Lancet, 2:851, 1986

Campbell S: The assessment of fetal development by diagnostic ultrasound. Clin Perinatal, 1:2,507, 1979

Fletcher JL: Update on pregnancy testing. Prin Care, 13:667, 1986

Glack L, Kulovich MV, Boner RC, et.al.: Diagnosis of respiratory distress syndrome by amniocentesis. Am J Obstet Gynecol, 109:440, 1971

Goldstein S: Vaginal endoscopy, Alan R Liss, New York, 1988

Rippey JH: Pregnancy tests: Evaluation and current status. CRC Crit Rev Clin Lab Sci, 19:353, 1984

Tabor A, Phillip J, Madsen M et al: Randomized controlled trials of genetic amniocentesis in 4606 low risk women. Lancet, 1:1287, 1986

BLEEDING DURING PREGNANCY

Cotton DB, Read JA, Paul RH et al: The conservative aggressive management of placenta praevia. Am J Obstet Gynecol, 137:687, 1980

Post D: Vasa praevia. Am J Obstet Gynecol, 104:151, 1979

Scott JR: Vaginal bleeding in the midtrimester of pregnancy. Am J Obstet Gynecol, 113:329, 1972

EXERCISE

Jimenez MH, Newton N: Activity and work during pregnancy and the postpartum period: A cross-cultural study of 202 societies. Am J Obstet Gynecol, 135:171, 1979

Lotgering FK, Gilbert RD, Longo LD: The interaction of exercise and pregnancy: A Review. Am J Obstet Gynecol, 149:560, 1989

NUTRITION

Begner L, Susser MW: Low birth weight and prenatal nutrition: An interpretive review. Pediatrics, 46:946, 1970

Fahey PJ, Boltri JM, Mark JS: Key issues on nutrition. From conception through infancy. Postgrad Med, 81:301, 1987

Hemminti E, Stanfield B: Routine administration of iron and vitamins during pregnancy: Review of controlled clinical trials. Br. J Obstet Gynecol, 85:404, 1978

Jarnfelt-Samisoe A: Nausea and vomiting in pregnancy. A review. Obstet Gynecol Surv, 42: 422, 1987

National Research Council: Alternative Dietary Practices and Nutritional Abuses during Pregnancy. Washington D.C. National Academy of Sciences, 1982

Piconce TA, Allen LH, Olsen PN, Fern MF: Pregnancy outcome in North American women. Ill effects of direct cigarette smoking, stress, and weight gain on placentas and on neonatal physical and behavioral characteristics. Am J Clin Nutr, 36:1214, 1982

WEIGHT GAIN

Abrams BF, Lans RK: Prepregnancy weight, weigh tgain and birth weight. Am J Obstet Gynecol, 154:503, 1986

Gormician A, Valentine L, Satter E: Relationship of maternal weight gain, prepregnancy weight and infant birth weight. J Am Diet Assoc, 77:662, 1980

LABOR AND BIRTH

Beazley JM: The active management of labor. Am J Obstet Gynecol, 122:161, 1975

Beck NC, Hall D: Natural childbirth: A review and analysis. Obstet Gynecol, 52:371, 1978

Capso AI: Force of labor. In Iffy L, Kaminetzky HA (eds.): Principles and Practice of obstetrics and perinatology, John Wiley & Sons, New York, 1981

Carlson JM, Diehl JA, Sachtleben-Murray M, et al: Maternal positioning during parturition in normal labor. Clin Obstet Gynecol, 30:83, 1987

Danforth DN, Buckingham JC, Roddick JW: Connective tissue changes incident to cervical effacement. Am J Obstet Gynecol, 80:939, 1960

Freidman EA, Sachtleben MR, Bresky PA: Dysfunctional labor. XXI. Longterm effects of labor and delivery on offspring: A matched pair analysis. Am J Obstet Gynecol, 150:941, 1984

Ulmsten U, Ueland K (eds.): The forces of labor: Uterine contractions and the resistance of the cervix. Clin Obstet Gynecol, 26:1. 1983

Whittle MJ, Miller FC: The evaluation of uterine activity. Am J Obstet Gynecol, 136:38, 1980

FORCEPS

Freidman EA, Sachtleben MR, Bresky PA: Dysfunctional labor. XXI. Longterm effects of labor and delivery on offspring: A matched pair analysis. Am J Obstet Gynecol, 150:941, 1984

Levine MG, Holroyde J, Woods JR, et al. Birth trauma: Incidence and predisposing factors. Obstet Gynecol, 63:792, 1984

McBride WG, Black BP, Brown CJ, et al. Method of delivery and development outcome at five years of age. Med J Aust, 1:301, 1979

Glossary

ABORTION – termination of a pregnancy. Broken into two categories: spontaneous abortion (miscarriage) is the termination of a pregnancy naturally by the body prior to the viability of the fetus. Hormonal, chromosomal anatomical and immunological abnormalities can trigger this type. An induced abortion is one in which unnatural means are used to terminate a pregnancy. This can be accomplished by either chemical or mechanical means.

ABRUPTIO PLACENTA – the partial or complete detachment of the placenta from the site of normal implantation at any time before the birth of the fetus.

ACQUIRED IMMUNE DEFICIENCY SYNDROME (AIDS) – As of 1993 more than 500,000 people have died from this disease. A disease that effects the entire immune system caused by the human immunodeficiency virus(HIV). A disease characterized by marked loss of T cells, thereby compromising the entire immune system. Secondary complications such as pneumocystis pneumonia are common. To date there is no known treatment or cure.

ALPHA-FETOPROTEIN – normal levels rise slowly during the entire pregnancy and peaks at about 30 weeks of gestation. A product of the fetal liver it is found in the fetal and maternal circulation as well as in the amniotic fluid. Levels of AFP in the maternal serum and in the amniotic fluid are generally elevated in the presence of neural tube defects. An elevated AFP does not necessarily mean NT defect nor does the absence of elevated levels mean there is no neurological defect as closed defects such as hydrocephalus will show no rise in AFP.

AMNIOCENTESIS – the aspiration of amniotic fluid for genetic screening purposes from the mother. Usually performed at 14-16 weeks, but becoming more common at 9-10 weeks. Performed under ultrasonic examination to determine proper needle placement. It has a spontaneous abortion rate of 0.1%.

AMNIOTIC BANDS – interruption of the amnion that cause adherence to the fetus and often times produces amputation of fetal limbs.

AMNIOTIC FLUID – a colorless fluid which fills the amniotic sac. At term it peaks at approximately 1000ml. It protects the fetus by providing a cushion, and temperature regulation for the fetus. The fluid as it presents at the opening of the cervix during labor also can provide what is known as a hydrostatic dilator.

AMNIOTIC FLUID EMBOLISM – when amniotic fluid enters the maternal circulation it can cause an embolism, and most often results in maternal death.

ANDROID PELVIS – not favorable for deliver as the inlet is heart-shaped with the fetal head having difficulty adapting itself to the triangular shape. The sidewalls converge.

ANENCEPHALY – the absence of a cranium and cerebral hemispheres. Not compatible with life.

ANTHROPOID PELVIS – the anterior-posterior diameter of the inlet exceeds the transverse diameter. Narrow side to side and long anterior to posterior, it is difficult for birth.

APGAR SCORE – a subjective measure of the well-being of the newborn which has been used since 1953 when it was introduced by a physician, Dr. Virginia Apgar. It is a qualitative test to determine the status of the newborn taken at 1 minute and 5 minutes. Rated are the heart rate, respiration, muscle tone, reflex irritability and color. Ten is a perfect score with the values of 0,1,or 2 being given to each character. Normally at one minute old, the child should have attained at least a score of 7, and at 5 minutes old the child should have attained a score of at least an 8. Children who have scores of 0-3 at five minutes tend to have a higher morbidity and mortality than those who have higher scores.

ASYNCLITISM – the lateral deflection of the fetal head toward the anterior or the posterior during a normal vertex birth.

BALLOTMENT – pushing up on the lower part of the uterus causes the fetus to float upward and then to come down and become palpable. This is thought to be a positive sign of pregnancy.

BARTHOLIN GLANDS – also known as the major vestibular glands, they are located at the vaginal opening. During sexual excitement these glands secrete a mucous-like substance.

BELLS PALSY – also known as facial paralysis. The 7th cranial nerve is effected. Usually occurring during the last trimester and the puerperium. It results most often in an unilateral pitosis of the eyelid and facial musculature. Subluxation of the cranial bones are often associated.

BRACHIAL NEURALGIA – pain in the neck, shoulder, or arm, that can radiate down to the fingers. It is due to nerve pressure or impingement at the level of the brachial plexus.

BRAXTON-HICKS CONTRACTIONS – intermittent, irregular and painless contractions of the uterus which begins during the end of the first trimester. Used as a probable sign of pregnancy.

BREECH PRESENTATION – the alignment of the fetus in the longitudinal pole where the buttock (frank breech), foot, lower extremity (incomplete breech) or the legs (complete breech).

BROW PRESENTATION – The fetal head is located in-between flexion and hyperextension. The presenting part is the head between the orbit and the anterior fontanelle.

CAPUT SUCCEDARUM – an edematous swelling of the scalp at the point of birth presentation.Resulting from interruption of the lymphatic supply to the scalp as in a brow or breech presentation

CARDINAL MOVEMENTS – a term used to describe the movements that occur during a normal labor: engagement, descent, flexion, internal rotation, and extension.

CEPHALOHEMATOMA – unilateral or bilateral pooling of blood between the periosteum and the underlying bone. Most often this pooling does not cross the suture line. Most frequently involving the parietal bones but can occur anywhere on the scalp.

CERVICAL DILATATION – the opening of the cervix during labor to permit the passage of the fetus. It is said to be completely dilated when it reaches 10 cm.

CERVIX – separates the isthmus of the uterus from the vagina. The cervical opening, the os, opens only for childbirth, or the expulsion of aborted or miscarried tissue

CESAREAN SECTION – the opening to the abdominal cavity and the uterus to allow birth to take place. It usually occurs under circumstances where normal vaginal birth is not possible. Most notable is the lack of cranial moulding.

CHADWICKS SIGN – mucous membranes of the vagina, vulva, and cervix become bluish-violet in color. This is thought to be a positive sign of pregnancy.

CHORIONIC VILLI SAMPLING – an alternative to amniocentesis, where a small portion of the chorion is sampled to detect fetal abnormalities. Performed either transvaginally or transcervically.

CLEFT PALATE (HARELIP) – a failure of fusion of the hard and soft palate in the newborn. Can occur for many genetic reasons as well as a result of pharmacological agents taken during pregnancy.

CLIMACTERIC – the time of life which marks the transition for a woman changing from a time of reproduction to a time of non-reproduction. In the U.S. the approximate age is around 51 years. The most prevalent and noticeable feature is the onset of menopause.

CLITORIS – located in the superior part of the vulva, and is analogous with the penis in the male. It is made up of three parts: 1) glans, 2) the body, and 3) two crura.

COCCYDYNIA – pain at the site of the coccyx bone. It can occur during the last trimester or after birth, or as a result of trauma during the non-pregnant state. It is most often caused by subluxation at the site.

COLOSTRUM – the yellow colored initial secretion from the breast for the first five days postpartum. Many antibodies and immunoglobulins have been found to be contained in this fluid, thus providing some immunological benefit to the child.

COMPOUND PRESENTATION – a part of the fetus is prolapsed alongside of the presenting part.

CONCEPTUS – all products of fertilization and conception including the embryo, fetus, membranes and placenta.

CONGENITAL HIP DISLOCATION – found very often in female neonates due to the presence of estrogen which allows the laxity of the ligaments of the femur to occur. Coupled with unusual positioning in utero.

CUSHINGS SYNDROME – initially described in 1912 by Harvey Cushing. Usually described as any excess or prolonged use by the body of glucocorticoids. The most common cause of the syndrome is excessive ACTH secretion by the pituitary resulting in hyperplasia of the adrenal glands. Signs and symptoms include obesity, moon face, purple cutaneous striae hypertension, and muscle wasting.

CYSTIC FIBROSIS – present in approximately 1 in 2,500 births, it is estimated that as many as 1 in 25 carry the gene for cystic fibrosis.

DE QUERVAIN TENDONITIS – swelling of the tendons located at the distal radius.

DYSTOCIA – abnormal labor divided into problems concerning the powers, the passage and the passenger.

ECTOPIC PREGNANCY – the Conceptus is located outside the endometrial cavity, with the most common site being the fallopian tubes. One (1) in eighty (80) pregnancies result in an ectopic. Signs and symptoms of this type of pregnancy are wide and diffuse with the most common being mild to severe pelvic pain of unknown origin.

EMBRYO – the fertilized mass once it has reached the uterus and is transformed from the blastocyst. The period of growth labeled "embryonic" lasts until week seven (7).

ENDOMETRIOSIS – the presence of endometrial tissues (uterine lining) outside the uterus. Suspected to be present in 20% of all women, it is postulated to be responsible for approximately 25% of all infertility. The most characteristic symptom is pelvic pain.

ENDOMETRIUM – the mucosal layer of the uterus.

ENDOMYOMETRITIS – an infection at the site of the placenta involving the decidua and adjacent myometrium. Most commonly caused by a bacterium.

ENGAGEMENT – the head of the fetus (its biparietal diameter) descends to a level below the pelvic inlet. Once the head has passed that level it is considered to be engaged.

EPIDURAL – a type of anesthesia used during labor. The epidural space is located in the vertebral column between the epidural sac in the anterior and the ligamentum flavum in the posterior. Ideally the anesthesia is administered through the interspace between the spinous processes. The advantages of this type of anesthesia is that it can be used for vaginal delivery or for a C-section if necessary.

EPISIOTOMY – the most common surgical procedure in obstetrics, it is the cutting of the perineum to allow the passage of the fetus. It can be either midline, or mediolateral. It is performed in lieu of allowing the perineum to tear risking full tear through the rectum.

ERYTHOBLASTOSIS FETALIS – hemolytic disease of the newborn caused by an incompatibility of the fetal and maternal blood. Can occur between an RH negative mother and an RH positive fetus.

ESTROGEN – the steroid hormone which is secreted by the ovarian follicle. It enters the endometrium by diffusion and allows the continuation of the corpus luteum. Increased in pregnancy, estrogen along with progesterone permits changes to the connective tissue which allows the fetus to grow within the woman's body.

EXTERNAL ELECTRONIC FETAL MONITORING – an ultrasound transducer is strapped on the outside of the mother's belly with an application of a coupling gel. The fetal heart rate is recorded directly onto a monitor where tracing can be examined.

EXTERNAL CONTRACTION MONITORING – used during high risk pregnancies to record the number and strength of contractions that occur during the latter stages of pregnancy. A displacement transducer is placed on the fundus of the mother and recordings are made periodically during the day.

ESTIMATED DATE OF CONFINEMENT (EDC) – the date the baby is due to be born averaging 266 days.

ESTROGEN REPLACEMENT THERAPY – estrogen derivatives prescribed to retard or cease the demineralization of bone after menopause. Studies have demonstrated that the loss of estrogen with the onset of menopause gives rise to the high incidence of fractures in postmenopausal women. The synthetic estrogen replacement can alter those changes. This type of therapy has also been linked to a high incidence of ovarian cancer in women who chose this type of therapy.

FACE PRESENTATION – the fetal head is hyper extended with occiput touching the back, and presenting part being the face between the orbit and the chin.

FERTILIZATION – the act of the sperm penetrating the egg and the contents of each mixing together.

FETUS – after the embryonic period (7 weeks) the growing embryo is given this term.

FISTULA – the abnormal connection between two passageways or two body areas which are normally separated by tissues. They occur most often as uterovaginal, vesicovaginal or urethovaginal.

GOODELL'S SIGN – softening of the cervix in pregnancy. Thought to be a positive sign of pregnancy.

GRASP REFLEX – the normal reflex found in the infant under the age of 6 months where the child will grab or grasp anything that is put into its hand. This is a normal reflex; up to that time. Beyond this age the child should have less of a closed hand and should make purpose-ful movements to grasp objects rather than reflexive movements.

GUILLAIN-BARRE SYNDROME – occurring most often following a viral disease such as mononucleosis, it is a progressive demyelinating disease. A significant number progress to the point of needing ventilatory assistance.

GYNECOID PELVIS – most common pelvic type in the female and is best suited for childbirth as the inlet is round or oval, with the transverse diameter slightly larger than the anterior-posterior diameter. The sidewalls are straight.

HEGAR'S SIGN – the palpable softening of the cervix during pregnancy. Thought to be a positive sign of pregnancy.

HUMAN CHORIONIC GONADOTROPIN (HCG) – a glycoprotein produced by the placenta. It will double every 2-3 days. This sharp increase in total amount lends itself to measurement and is used as the primary measure of pregnancy and gestation.

HYDATIDIFORM MOLE – (molar pregnancy) characterized by abnormalities of the chorionic villi. A complete HM is seen when there is little or no development of the fetal sacs. The chromosomal composition very often is 46XX completely of paternal origin, signifying the fact that the duplication of genetic material occurred only with the sperm. Occasionally this is not true. In an incomplete HM there is some formation of sacs at least the formation of the amniotic sac. The chromosomal composition of this type of mole is 69XXX or 69XXY. Again, this type demonstrates the presence of two paternal complements. There is a slight risk of these types of pregnancies becoming a choriocarcinoma, and must be followed.

HYDRAMNIOS – an excess of amniotic fluid.

HYMEN – or vaginal opening is comprised of elastic and collagenous connective tissue. During first intercourse the hymen is opened completely, and some tearing may occur. In past times this presence of tearing was a sign of the lack of virginity. In active modern women, the hymen can be torn early in life with little or no bleeding or telltale signs.

HYPERBILIRUBINEMIA – an increase in bilirubin resulting in jaundice. Most commonly treated with hydration and an ultraviolet lamp.

HYPEREMESIS GRAVIDARUM – also known as morning sickness. Beginning in the third trimester and most often ends during the second trimester. Most often a benign condition, but can lead to dehydration and ultimate death if not contained. Its causes have long been speculated upon, but known to be caused by the hormonal changes of pregnancy especially the increase in production of estrogen and progesterone.

IN VITRO FERTILIZATION (IVF-ET) – the fertilization of the egg by the sperm outside of the uterus with transfer of the viable embryo to the uterus.

INFERTILITY – the failure of the basic processes of human production. The basis of the failure ranges from physical to the emotional to the psychological. It does not imply sterility which is an irreversible condition.

INTERNAL ELECTRONIC FETAL MONITORING – the heartbeat of the fetus is measured by boring an electrode into the fetal scalp. A metal piece of the monitor serves as a second pole and the sodium rich vaginal fluids create a salt bridge whereby the electrical voltage difference between the two electrodes can be measured.

INTERNATIONAL CHILDBIRTH EDUCATION ASSOCIATION (ICEA) – an international association dedicated to practical education with respect to childbirth. Their motto is: "Freedom of Choice through Knowledge of Alternatives".

KYPHOSIS – the normal anterior to posterior convex curve found in the thoracic region of the normal healthy adult spine.

LABOR – the physiological process whereby sustained, painful and regular contractions of increasing frequency and strength cause progressive effacement and dilatation of the cervix and ultimate expulsion of the fetus. In the primagravida, the duration is approximately 14 hours and in the multigravida 7-9 hours. Often labor is broken down into the power (uterine contraction), passage (the bony pelvis and surrounding soft tissue) and the passenger (the fetus).

LABIA MAJORA – two round folds of adipose tissue that extend from the mons pubis to the posterior fusion with the perineum. The posterior site is called the posterior commissure. This structure is analogous with the male scrotum.

LABIA MINORA – located under the labia majora, their size and shape vary widely. In the nulliparous woman they are seen only when the majora are separated. In the multiparous woman, they occasionally hang below the majora.

LEOPOLD – a systematic series of maneuvers totaling four in all which determine the fetal position. Should an abnormal position such as a breech become discovered as a result of the leopolds maneuver then a version is likely to be needed to change the position of the child.

LEUKORRHEA – vaginal discharge in the pregnant woman which is most often increased in amount.

LOCHIA – the early vaginal discharge of the puerperium. After the first few days when bleeding is still present it is known as lochia rubra. After 5 days the bleeding gradually remits and the discharge becomes paler, and is then known as lochia serosa. After 20 or 12 days, it becomes more white in color due to its content of leukocytes and is known as lochia alba.

LORDOSIS – the normal anterior to posterior concave curve found in the lumbar and cervical regions of the normal healthy adult spine.

LYME DISEASE – caused by the spirochete borrelia burgdorferi. Characterized by a bulls-eye lesion at the site of the tick bite, followed by migratory arthalgia, an erythema that is chronic and migratory. The most common symptoms resemble the flu.

MCDONALD'S SIGN – the uterine body and the cervix can be flexed upon one another. Thought to be a positive sign of pregnancy.

MECONIUM ASPIRATION SYNDROME – acute trauma to the fetus in utero causes the passage of meconium. Fetal aspiration of the amniotic fluid filled with meconium can cause an obstruction of the upper respiratory tract.

MECONIUM STAINING – the amniotic fluid is stained with fetal fecal contents. It has traditionally been regarded as a sign of fetal distress. It remains unknown as to why it occurs but its presence may not always be due to fetal distress. In general, the fetal mortality rate is increased in the presence of meconium as well as lowered Apgar scores.

MENOPAUSE – the cessation of physiological uterine bleeding which marks the beginning of climacteric.

MENSTRUATION – the cyclical discharge of blood, mucous and debris from the uterus. Occurring in a cycle that varies around 28 days, it begins (menarche) at approximately the age of 9-10 and ends during menopause at approximately the 4th or 5th decade of life. In between it can also stop due to pregnancy, lactation, and abnormal stress.

MIDWIFERY – from the Old English mid meaning with, and wif meaning wife or woman. The word midwife was used as early as the 13th and 14th century.

MONS PUBIS – also known as the mons veneris, is the fatty covering over the symphysis pubis. The mons is covered with the hair that is known as the escutcheon.

MORO REFLEX – clapping, jerking, or any sudden movements performed around the child. A normal response under the age of 6 months is abduction of the arms, extension of the elbows, wrist and fingers, followed by adduction of the arms and flexion of the elbows, arms, and fingers. If this persists long after 6 months of age it may be considered pathological.

MORULA – the fertilized egg which has divided into 16 or more cells.

MULTIPARA – a woman who has given birth to two or more fetuses. It can also be considered as the number of fetuses to reach viability.

MULTIPARITY – a term used to denote a woman who has had three or more children

MYOMETRIUM – the major portion of the uterus which is comprised of smooth muscle and connective tissue.

NABOTHIAN CYSTS – occlusion of the ducts of the cervical glands.

NAGELE'S RULE – the mean duration of pregnancy is approximately 266 days. Since the exact time of conception is most often unknown, it's often measured from the first day of the last menstruation, add seven days, subtract three months and add one year to determine the due date or the estimated date of confinement (EDC).

NOTOCHORD – the center of the growing embryo is known as the primitive streak. It is from this primitive streak that the notochord arises. The remnants of the notochord are the nucleus pulposus of the intervertebral discs.

NULLIGRAVIDA – a woman who has never been pregnant.

NULLIPARA – a woman who has never completed a pregnancy.

OBSTETRICS – derived from the word in Latin, osbsterix, meaning midwife.

OBSTETRICAL CONJUGATE – the distance between the sacral promentory and the symphysis pubis.

OBSTETRIC PALSY – a catchall term used to denote any type of nonspecific neurological condition found in pregnancy or the postpartum period.

OLIGOHYDRAMNIOS – a decrease in the volume of amniotic fluid.

ORTILANI – an orthopedic check where a positive finding is a click. The knee is flexed and the hip joint externally rotated. Under normal circumstances the movement at the acetabulum is smooth and without an audible clicking sound. When a click is heard this is considered a positive finding and an indication of a possible congenital hip dysplasia.

OSTEOPOROSIS – the state where a bone or bones have lost sufficient matrix so as to become predisposed to fracture. Broken down into two categories: primary: (senile) accompanies age and often menopause in women. Most often affects women age 55-70, and affects the longbones of the arms and hips; secondary: mineral loss and often accompanying fracture due to disease, and/or specific drug use.

OTITIS MEDIA – middle ear infection which can be broken down into two categories 1) acute or purulent, 2) chronic or serious. It is the most common illness in children under the age of three years and accounts for the majority of sick visits to the pediatrician

OVARIES – small almond shaped organs which house and mature the ova. In addition they synthesize and secrete steroid hormones

PARACERVICAL – anesthetics are injected at the outer rim of the cervix through a transvaginal injection. Due to the fact that the local injection may lead to fetal complications this type of anesthetics is not often used.

PARTURIENT – a woman who is presently in labor.

PASSAGEWAY – the bony pelvis and soft tissue through which the fetus must pass during delivery.

PASSENGER – the fetus.

PELVIC INFLAMMATORY DISEASE (PID) – inflammation often caused by sexually transmitted disease. It is estimated that 25% of all reproductive women will have at least one bout of PID during her reproductive life.

PELVIC INLET – the pelvic area bounded anteriorly by the symphysis pubis, laterally by the linea terminalis of the ishium, and posteriorly by the sacral promentory and the ala.

PELVIC OUTLET – the pelvic area made up of two triangles. The anterior triangle is formed by the area underneath the pubic arch. The posterior triangle is formed by the tip of the sacrum, the two ishial tuberosities and the sacrosciatic ligaments.

PELVIMETRY – measurement of the bony pelvis to determine the ability of the fetus to pass through during the birth process. Measurements are the obstetric conjugate - the anterior to posterior diameter, and the diagonal conjugate which is the diagonal measurement of the opening.

At one time these measurements were taken from X-ray analysis which is done only in rare instances now.

PERINEUM – made up from the pelvic diaphragm: coccygeal and levator ani muscles, as well as the urogenital diaphragm: deep transverse perineal muscles, and urethral constrictor, and the internal and external fascia.

PHENYLKETONURIA – an autosomal recessive disorder which is characterized as an inborn error of metabolism. It is due to a decrease in phenylalanine hydroxylase activity resulting in an inability to convert phenylalanine to tyrosine.

PICA – the ingestion in a compulsive manner of nonfood substances with little or no nutritive value in response to a lack of nutrients in the pregnant body. It is not limited to pregnancy.

PISKACEK'S SIGN – the uterus becomes asymmetrical once implantation has taken place. The well-defined soft prominence of the cornu at the side of implantation. Thought to be a positive sign of pregnancy.

PLACENTA ACCRETA – the abnormal adherence of the placenta to the uterine wall.

PLACENTA PRAEVIA – condition where the placenta is located in the lower pole of the uterus where a part of placenta precedes the presenting part of the fetus. If the placenta covers the os, the C-section may need to occur.

PLATYPELLOID PELVIS – least common, also known as a flat pelvis.

POSTERIOR COMMISURE – the area where the labia majora fuse with the perineum.

POWERS – the uterine contractions during labor which expel the fetus.

PROGESTERONE – a steroid hormone which mediates the action of estrogen. Together with estrogen, it also increases in pregnancy and allows alteration in the connective tissue of the pregnant woman's body.

PREMENSTRUAL SYNDROME – repeat symptoms which occur on a monthly basis which affect mood and behavior. Traditionally attributed to large secretions and subsequent withdrawal of progesterone.

PRIMIPARA – a woman who has given birth to only one fetus.

PUERPERA – a woman who has just given birth. She is considered to be in this stage for approximately 12 weeks.

PSEUDOCYESIS – imaginary pregnancy. Occurs in women who have a deep desire to be pregnant or in women nearing menopause.

QUICKENING – the perception of fetal movement by the mother, usually felt initially during the 16th-18th week. The absence of this may signal fetal demise.

RESPIRATORY DISTRESS SYNDROME TYPE II – (transient tachypnea of the newborn) usually seen in the full term neonate, and is seen at birth or shortly after and is characterized by retraction of the lungs, tachypnea and grunting. Diagnosed with the help of X-ray where the lungs are over-inflated, with flattening of the diaphragm. This type of respiratory distress resolves in 1-5 days.

RESPIRATORY DISTRESS SYNDROME (RDS/HYALINE MEMBRANE DISEASE)– occurring only in the premature infant and is due to the immaturity of the adult pathway production of surfactant. Surfactant allows the lungs to expand normally. This type of respiratory syndrome has a high incidence of mortality and morbidity.

ROOMING IN – the hospital, or birthing center model whereby the newborn and mother share the same room. This bypasses the use of the nursery.

SCIATIC NEURALGIA – inflammation of the sciatic nerve or nerve roots at the level of the lumbar plexus or at the level of the sciatic notch of the ilium. This is most often due in pregnancy to the hormonal as well as structural changes that occur.

SHOULDER DYSTOCIA – in the postdate fetus the shoulder blocks the passageway, and the fetus is unable to pass necessitating a C-section.

SHOULDER PRESENTATION – The fetus's lie perpendicular to the long axis of the mother, also known as a transverse lie.

SIMIAN CREASE – a continuous horizontal palmar crease seen in certain conditions such a Downs Syndrome

STERILITY – incapable of bearing young or of viable reproduction.

TALIPES EQUINOVARUS – also known a clubfoot. It is the extreme inversion of the foot usually due to extreme positioning in utero.

TELOGEN EFFLUVIUM – a self-limiting condition seen postpartum where a woman has spontaneous hair loss. It usually begins at 1-4 months postpartum and lasts from 4-12 months.

TOXIC SHOCK SYNDROME – an acute illness caused by staphylococcus aureus. Characterized by high fever, diffuse rash, desquamation of the skin, vomiting, diarrhea. Associated most closely with menstruation and tampon use.

TRACHEOESOPHAGEAL FISTULA – segmental atresia of the esophagus resulting in a blind pouch in the upper tract. The lower tract then communicates with the upper trachea or a bronchus through a connecting tube or fistula

UTERUS – the muscular internal organ of pregnancy. The internal covering is comprised of endometrium. It is comprised of three parts: 1) the body, 2) the isthmus and 3) the cervix. It normally varies in size from 6-10 cm, depending upon the parity of the woman.

ULTRASOUND – the electric stimulation of a piezoelectric crystal which produces high frequency energy that is reflected from solid and fluid structures in the body. These reflections are then translated into an image. These images are used to detect gynecological abnormalities as well as abnormal conditions of pregnancy. Fetal measurements, placental placement, fetal condition, and overall anatomical survey can be performed. In addition to the visual pictures, blood flow can be measured by means of ultrasonic measurement by Doppler which measured moving targets.

UMBILICAL CORD PROLAPSE – the umbilical cord falls down alongside of the presenting part during birth.

VACUUM EXTRACTION – the use of a suctioning device as a vacuum attached to the head in the vertex presentation to aid in the delivery of the fetus.

VAGINA – the connection from the vulva to the uterus. It is the organ of sexual intercourse, and the conduit of uterine material. It carries the contents of the menses as well as the fetus during birth. In the anterior its membranes are in contact with the bladder, and in the posterior, its membranes are in contact with the rectum. Occasionally, these membranes become ruptured and abnormal connections are made.

VASA PREVIA – the rupture of a fetal vessel.

VERSION – the movement of the fetus externally to change a breech presentation to a cephalic presentation. Done approximately during the 36th-37th week, under real-time ultrasound. The examiner will rotate an unengaged fetus from the breech to the cephalic.

Index

A

B

C

D

E

F

G

H

I

K

L

M

N

O

P

Q

R

S

T

U

V

W